The Restless Compendium

Felicity Callard • Kimberley Staines • James Wilkes
Editors

The Restless Compendium

Interdisciplinary Investigations of Rest and Its Opposites

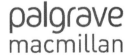
palgrave
macmillan

Editors
Felicity Callard
Durham University, Durham
United Kingdom

Kimberley Staines
Durham University, Durham
United Kingdom

James Wilkes
Durham University, Durham
United Kingdom

ISBN 978-3-319-45263-0   ISBN 978-3-319-45264-7 (ebook)
DOI 10.1007/978-3-319-45264-7

Library of Congress Control Number: 2016951673

Cover pattern: © Melisa Hasan

Printed on acid-free paper

This Palgrave Macmillan imprint is published by Springer Nature
The registered company is Springer International Publishing AG
The registered company address is: Gewerbestrasse 11, 6330 Cham, Switzerland

FOREWORD

I start this foreword with a deceptively simple question: What difference might it make doing research in public? This was one of the key challenges faced by the first inhabitants of Wellcome Collection's Hub, located as they have been in the capital of a thriving public venue. The brave and brilliantly experimental Hubbub team have spent two years (and roughly £1 million) living out one possible answer.

Four features of their model stand out: they have fixed on and then refined an intriguing topic; selected and energetically mixed an eclectic range of investigators; tested and refined effective ways of working together; and finally, they have skilfully integrated modes of investigation with others of dissemination. Interestingly, these are also core attributes of the curatorial practices that Wellcome Collection has elaborated since opening in 2007. It is not too surprising maybe that investigation-led programming bears striking methodological resemblances to research conducted with the public in mind.

Defined in their own carefully chosen words, Hubbub has been concerned with the 'dynamics of rest, noise and work'. We live in frantic times when many of us measure our worth according to how busy we seem, but we are simultaneously worried sick by the consequences. When is it healthy to be turbulent or calm, noisy or still, and for whom? There are urgent questions here, but luckily the topics to which Hubbub has chosen to apply a cross-curricular mindset are also intrinsically fascinating: the experience and psychological characteristics of mind wandering; people's movements across the city; and current practices of unemployment, which can ironically turn into a form of exhausting busyness.

One invention of our frantically busy era is the strapline: a snappy phrase that people in a rush can catch on the move. Established a decade ago, Wellcome Collection initially identified its essence in the juxtaposition of three common words: medicine, life and art. A decade of adventurous exhibitions and events delving into this conceptual triangle has taught us just how much more intriguing (not to mention easier) it is to start in the middle (with life): considering, for example, twins rather than genetics. Hubbub has also been, it seems, instinctively drawn to a topic infused with common currency, which offers a handle that non-experts can grasp. 'The opposites of rest' is a provocative notion that can be approached in many ways and that demands interstitial thinking: an idea not exclusively owned by one discipline. Crucially, this has also turned out to be a stranger proposition than it first appeared, revealing surprising unknowns amongst what was already known.

Even the most compelling and approachable subject would remain dormant without the right mix of disciplined adventurers ready to bring it to life. In Hubbub's case they arrived in the form of researchers from across the campus, as well as artists, broadcasters and public engagement professionals. A common denominator running through their inventive investigations of sub-topics such as stress, noise, the voice, work and sound has been the active integration of insights into subjective experiences of medicine (often couched in terms of intensely personal meanings understood from within) combined with more objective versions of the human condition emerging from biomedical laboratories and statistical analyses, where phenomena are explained from without.

Enthusiastic rhetoric that boosts interdisciplinary activity abounds these days; so much fresh thinking seems to be emerging from those who dare to forage beyond subject specialisms. Within an academic framework this is still a profoundly unnatural activity, and with good reason. In the late eighteenth century, Albrecht von Haller was already pointing out that universities derived much of their effectiveness precisely from dividing 'the sciences into small parts [which gave] each man a small and limited responsibility'.[i] His observation was prophetic: the number of university-based fields of investigation multiplied some tenfold during the twentieth century – a tree of knowledge from which much of what we know about the world today emerged.

---

[i] Quoted from Peter Burke, *A Social History of Knowledge: From the Encyclopedie to Wikipedia*, vol. 2 (Cambridge: Polity, 2012), 160.

The more mature elaboration of disciplines did clearly throw up barriers to uncovering new insights, with bigger pictures in research being overlooked. But while positive regard for interdisciplinary work is almost ubiquitous, we seem to know surprisingly little about how such projects actually work, and why they don't when they fail. One of the great legacies of Hubbub's two-year residency lies in the group's attentive introspection, as well as the generous eagerness of the researchers to share what has been discovered about just how much discipline needs to be applied to foster creative interdisciplinarity.

As Hubbub members eloquently testify, where these unusual investigative activities actually happen (the physical spaces) has been a vital part of their project too. The Hub was deliberately designed as a dynamic working environment that should take maximum advantage of the lower public floors: a place from which to observe and then embrace the intriguing company of strangers who populate them – sometimes as subjects, sometimes as collaborators, sometimes as audiences and often indistinguishably as all three. The public realm, it turns out, provides an ideal 'neutral' territory, where people are mostly ignorant of every specialism except their own, and in which a rather rigid disciplinary matrix can artfully be folded back in on itself.

Hubbub would be the last to claim that it has cracked the one way in which to do it, but its has been an inventive and highly productive experiment in public research which many will follow.

Ken Arnold
Creative Director, Wellcome Trust

ACKNOWLEDGEMENTS

We thank all those in London, Durham and elsewhere who have worked with us to bring Hubbub to life. We are grateful to Charles Fernyhough and Claudia Hammond, Associate Directors of Hubbub, for their advice, feedback and contributions to this book.

We also thank The Pioneer Health Foundation for kind permission to reproduce the image and unpublished material in Chap. 10: 'Mother watches while she and her daughter have their tea', Wellcome Library Archive, SA/PHC/H.1/6/8; Innes Hope Pearse, 'Medical Considerations for the Control of Contraception', p. 4, Wellcome Library Archive, SA/PHC/E.16/1, copyright The Pioneer Health Foundation.

This work was supported by the Wellcome Trust [103817/Z/14/Z], which also enabled us to publish this book in Open Access.

CONTENTS

LIST OF FIGURES

LIST OF TABLES

CHAPTER 1

Introduction

Felicity Callard, Kimberley Staines and James Wilkes

Abstract In this introduction, editors Felicity Callard, Kimberley Staines and James Wilkes describe the problem of rest – a ubiquitous concept whose presence or absence affects people, in different ways, everywhere. Depending on whether one is working clinically, historically, artistically, scientifically or through political and economic analysis, 'rest' has many looks and feels. The complexities of investigating such a phenomenon gave rise to Hubbub, the project out of which this edited book emerged. The editors describe how the book draws on research and practice undertaken during Hubbub's two-year residency in The Hub at Wellcome Collection. They outline the book's organizing structure, which groups the work of social scientists, scientists, humanities scholars, artists and broadcasters by scale of investigation, into minds, bodies and practices.

Keywords Experiment · Interdisciplinarity · Rest · Restless · Rhythm

Rest is a ubiquitous concept. Its presence or absence, its qualities and how it functions affect everyone, everywhere. Defining rest is problematic:

F. Callard (✉) · K. Staines · J. Wilkes
Durham University, Durham, United Kingdom
e-mail: felicity.callard@durham.ac.uk; staines.kimberley@gmail.com; wilkes_ja@yahoo.co.uk

F. Callard et al. (eds.), *The Restless Compendium*,
DOI 10.1007/978-3-319-45264-7_1

1

both its meaning and what it looks and feels like are affected by many and various socio-political, economic and cultural factors. Our struggles with and against rest are deeply personal: some of us seek to find it, interpreting that desire as a need for peace and stillness, while others find themselves forced to take rest without desiring to, entering into a strange circumstance in which others perceive their 'rest' entirely differently from how they perceive it themselves.

To counter the difficulty of defining rest, we have looked elsewhere to see what might constitute 'restlessness', or 'unrest' – the opposites of rest, if you will. Key areas have emerged: work and activity, noise and sound, mental restiveness and tumult. But what happens if these opposites are sometimes deemed restful by those who experience them? Can interpretations of rest and unrest be universal? And what is it that we are actually *doing* when we're resting? These are not idle speculations: rest brings with it serious questions about public health and wellbeing, about the conditions under which rest, work and activity can be considered restorative or pathological, for which social groups and at which historical times.

Consistently, we have found the boundary of what constitutes rest to shift and reshape, according to who is doing the investigating. The phenomenon of rest, in light of its complex physiological, clinical, political-economic and aesthetic properties, demands an interdisciplinary investigation which can challenge commonly held assumptions. It was from such a demand that Hubbub was born.

Hubbub is a research project consisting of a network of researchers and practitioners operating in the fields of mental health, the neurosciences, the arts, humanities, social sciences and public engagement. We collaborate to unpick, remake and transform what is meant by rest and its opposites. The group made a successful bid for Wellcome Trust funding in early 2014, receiving the inaugural Hub Award, a £1 million grant funding a two-year residency in The Hub. This is a new, purpose-built space on the fifth floor of Wellcome Collection, in the heart of London, designed to facilitate and support collaborative interdisciplinary research. Written at the end of our two-year residency, this book gathers a selection of short essays from Hubbub collaborators, describing aspects of our research into rest as it has happened so far. *The Restless Compendium* aims, in teasing out the ambiguity and complexity of rest, to prompt thought by opening up perspectives that might not ordinarily be considered directly related to this theme, and to open up pathways for further conversations.

The book is organized into three sections: Minds, Bodies and Practices. This division does not imply any categorical separation between these three; rather, it identifies a shared centre of gravity for the essays within each section, allowing readers to better navigate shared thematics. For example, while many of the essays grouped under 'Minds' also deal with the body or with cultural practices, we have chosen to group them according to their common focus on thoughts, interiority and subjective experiences.

This structure allows us to organize the book by scales of enquiry rather than discipline, expertise or historical period, moving from the subjective and personal to the interpersonal and culturally embedded. There are moments within this trajectory where individual essays collapse or interrupt this rule-of-thumb, but this method of grouping allows us to fulfil an interdisciplinary imperative of bringing multiple approaches and discourses into juxtaposition, rendering visible their sometimes covert connections. It allows us to set practice-based research alongside more traditional modes of scholarly enquiry, to create a hybrid space in which to address some of the topics that have exercised us over the last two years.

Nevertheless, we are aware that one reader's bracing variety is another's hopeless muddle, and we have thought carefully about how to keep this compendium on the right side of chaos, and how to create tools for readers seeking to follow themes across the book. One such tool, we hope, is this introduction, which draws out salient threads across the sections. Another tool is the further reading many contributors have provided to close their essays – pointers to those who want to investigate particular issues in greater depth. A third is the abstract immediately preceding each chapter, which provides a précis not only of chapter content but of how the work emerged from the wider collaborative Hubbub project. A fourth lies within the body of the essays themselves, where points of particular resonance are picked out with cross-references to other chapters in the compendium.

'Minds' focuses on subjective, inner experiences. The topic of mind wandering has been a focus of interest for Hubbub, as a state which is neither properly active (in the sense of directed and controlled) nor properly at rest (given the intense activity that states like daydreaming engender).

Three chapters in this section approach this topic from differing historical perspectives, ranging from medieval Christian writings (Chap. 3) to modern accounts in the human sciences and in fiction (Chaps. 4 and 5). They examine how daydreaming intersects with contemporary neuroscientific concepts such as the default mode network (Chap. 2) and describe descriptive experience sampling (DES), a psychological method for obtaining rich phenomenological data about inner experience (Chap. 6). The linguistic aspect of mind wandering is further explored when DES is used to examine the relationship between language, experience and attention in poetry (Chap. 7). The significance of language in structuring subjective experiences of rest also informs Chap. 8, which presents initial findings from The Rest Test, our global survey which asked participants questions on their resting habits and subjective responses to rest, as well as deploying psychological scales.

The chapters in 'Bodies' examine how particular individuals and collectives are called into being and organized around questions of rest and its opposites. Throughout the section, considerable interplay takes place between somatic, mental and social states, as in Chap. 9, which explores attempts to produce relaxation through specific bodily disciplines throughout the twentieth century. In Chap. 10, a parallel historical moment in interwar London is excavated through fiction informed by the archives of the 'Peckham Experiment', where bodies were configured around particular ideas of vitality and health. This speaks to a concern about the city and its potential to mutually shape and be shaped by bodies – a concern shared by two chapters (Chaps. 11 and 12) – which think about and gather data on social, rather than individual, bodily rhythms of rest and restlessness. Chapters about lullabies and the practice of drawing (Chaps. 14 and 13) both underline the role of the dynamic body, gendered or abstracted to a pencil point, in producing culture, knowledge or the possibility of resistance. Chapters 15 and 16 take the phenomenon of autonomous sensory meridian response (ASMR), a feeling of tingly relaxation which would seem to be primarily somatic, and consider it from complementary psychological and linguistic perspectives.

'Practices' opens up questions of how, why and when certain ways of being or working are construed as appropriately or inappropriately restful. The section begins with an exploration of how the dynamics of rest and lack of rest can be experienced vividly through sound, both in musical composition (Chap. 17) and through building and using devices to measure the noise impact of living under the Heathrow Airport flight path in London (Chap. 18). The consideration of dynamics moves beyond the sounded to the social in Chap. 19, which describes an experiment ('In The Diary Room') that gathers material on the rhythms and energies of Hubbub's own collaborative work. How social inequality affects both work and rest becomes pressingly visible in Chap. 21, which comprises a dialogue about collaborative work undertaken with men who live in a homeless hostel, and about the impact of government benefits policies on their lives. Politics are equally at play in a consideration of the invisibility of affective and other kinds of labour in the context of our own research project (Chap. 20). Attitudes towards work lead us to contemplate representations of laziness and sloth in literature in Chap. 22, before an artist working to a deadline races to complete work and down tools before Shabbat, the 'day of rest', begins (Chap. 23).

Interconnecting themes can be found between chapters in all three sections. One example we propose is the theme of *experiment*, which would draw together the scientific use of DES and its deployment as an experimental poetic tool (Chaps. 6 and 7 in 'Minds'); critical-creative experiments in artists' practices, ranging from interventions in the genre of the lullaby to engagements with the performance underway in an ASMR role-play (Chaps. 14 and 16 in 'Bodies'); and the experimental assemblages of a stochastic musical composition or the 'In the Diary Room' study, which gathers unscripted video data from the inhabitants of our shared working space (Chaps. 17 and 19 in 'Practices'). Other ways of clustering contributions to the book might be via materials and data, politics, historical periods, disciplines, genres or modes of address. We invite the reader to explore the book, plotting own path through the sections, perhaps inspired by these suggested themes, and hopefully discovering shared themes of own. In doing so, we hope the reader will be exposed to new methodologies and be able to explore how different practices (including musical composition, political activism, literary fiction and scientific experimentation) can allow for different ways of interpreting and interrogating research questions.

Our compendium takes seriously its genre: it comprises condensed representations of larger bodies of research and practice. As such, it functions as a series of snapshots of what we, as Hubbub, have been thinking about and doing, singly and collaboratively, during our residency. Our volume does not attempt to address the full scope of topics, problems, issues and actors that gather around the term rest. Hubbub's experimental make-up encouraged collaborators to develop work in whichever direction they saw fit. This had the effect of prizing open certain areas of enquiry likely not at the forefront of most people's minds when thinking about rest and its opposites. Our aliveness to serendipity has allowed the terrain of rest on which we have been working to shift in unexpected and, we believe, productive ways. That we have worked as much on mind wandering as we have on mindfulness serves, we hope, to recalibrate some of the normative assumptions that we – and perhaps you – make in relation to what is restful and what is not.

We acknowledge that our tendency to wander down particular alleys rather than others leaves some paths tracked only lightly, or not at all. In many respects, our concerns have been extensive. The Rest Test is a global survey; Hubbub has been preoccupied with ferocious transformations in the governance of worklessness, unemployment and housing; and the tools that collaborators have piloted have the potential to be taken up by a wide variety of actors. But we want, nonetheless, to emphasize our partialness and, in some important respects, our 'provinciality'. That most of our research and practice has emerged from, or been grounded in, a European and North American, and a predominantly monolingual context – with all the grounding assumptions that brings – only serves to spur us, in future work, to disrupt the models, concepts and starting points that we use when thinking about rest. We are acutely aware of the need for additional sociological, anthropological and historical research that would be better able to attend to all the differences that class, ethnicity, geographical and geopolitical location, debility and disability make to the experience, and very definitions, of rest and its opposites.

As our collective work has developed – and as we consider the data from our Rest Test – we have become even more aware of how unevenly rest is distributed, as well as of those voices and bodies that are occluded by dominant discourses about rest and noise. We have also become interested in what happens if one shifts the central premise of this phase of work. In other words, we want to think about the implications of moving away from the sometimes static dyad of rest/opposites of rest, and making that dyad dynamic. Rhythm – like rest – does work physiologically, phenomenologically, clinically and aesthetically, and we anticipate this being a substantial focus of our future work. You might, then, choose to read this compendium as much through attending to its rhythms and dynamics as through looking for, and listening to, the work of noise and silence.

Felicity Callard is Director of Hubbub and an academic at Durham University (Department of Geography and Centre for Medical Humanities). Her interdisciplinary research focuses on the history and present of psychiatry, psychology, psychoanalysis and the neurosciences. She is co-author of *Rethinking Interdisciplinarity Across the Social Sciences and Neurosciences* (Palgrave Macmillan, 2015).

Kimberley Staines is Project Coordinator of Hubbub and is employed by Durham University (Department of Geography). She has a background in law and publishing; is a Master's student in Psychosocial Studies at Birkbeck, University of London; and is a trustee of a food bank in London.

James Wilkes is an Associate Director of Hubbub. He is a poet and writer, as well as a researcher at Durham University (Department of Geography). His interests range across contemporary and modernist poetry, audio and visual art, and their intersections with the life sciences.

PART I

Minds

CHAPTER 2

Altered States: Resting State and Default Mode as Psychopathology

Ben Alderson-Day and Felicity Callard

Abstract Psychologist Ben Alderson-Day and geographer Felicity Callard share an interest in understanding how interdisciplinary approaches to the brain sciences that involve the social sciences and humanities can help open up new research questions and methods through which to understand pathological and non-pathological states of mind. Both have been interested in the fertility of resting-state research paradigms and the default mode network in this regard. Ben has collaborated on novel experimental investigations of inner experience during the resting state, and Felicity has focused on how tracing historical antecedents of resting-state research might reorient certain current scientific assumptions.

Keywords Autism · Default mode network · fMRI · Psychopathology · Psychosis · Resting state

Resting-state functional magnetic resonance imaging research (rsfMRI) investigates spontaneously or intrinsically generated neural activity. While this rapidly expanding field is a recent one – extending back only across the last two decades – attempts to understand what the brain and mind are doing while 'at rest' have a significantly longer history. The human

B. Alderson-Day (✉) · F. Callard
Durham University, Durham, United Kingdom
e-mail: benjamin.alderson-day@durham.ac.uk; felicity.callard@durham.ac.uk

© The Author(s) 2016
F. Callard et al. (eds.), *The Restless Compendium*,
DOI 10.1007/978-3-319-45264-7_2

sciences have made many attempts to position the human body in particular ways so as to elicit what the mind does when it is not overly preoccupied with responding to external stimuli. In 1930, for example, Hans Berger, in one of his early reports on the use of the electroencephalogram (EEG) in humans, described 'completely relaxed' experimental subjects who 'lay comfortably and with eyes closed on a couch which was insulated from the surrounding by glass feet'.[1]

Resting-state fMRI follows on the heels of such attempts: the 'at rest' condition involves the experimental participant being asked to lie still and relax, either with eyes closed or with eyes open while fixating on a cross.[2] But this research has also extensively reconfigured assumptions about the working of the brain. In particular, the demonstration that the brain shows a consistent pattern of activation – the 'default mode' – during 'rest' has challenged scientific understandings (from metabolic, cellular and psychological perspectives) about the ways in which a resting body might be accompanied by a distinctly 'restless' brain and mind.

The default mode network (DMN) – a network consistently activated during the 'default mode' – refers to a set of brain regions that tend to show synchronized brain activity when the brain is not engaged in an explicit task. The idea of 'default' derives largely from the observation that these areas (primarily medial prefrontal cortex, posterior cingulate/precuneus, and lateral parietal cortex) tend to deactivate in response to external psychological tasks, indicating 'a heretofore-unrecognized organization within the brain's intrinsic or on-going activity'.[3] Increased activity of these regions during periods of so-called 'rest' has suggested the importance of introspective processes such as mind wandering, daydreaming and self-reflection.[i] In this way, the 'default' of the DMN has historically been defined as the flip side of a range of focused, controlled and externally oriented processes: an image in negative of the aware and externally attentive brain.[4]

These attempts to characterize the brain and mind 'at rest' raise complex problems about how one constitutes a 'baseline', and the extent to which a resting state holds consistency in and across individuals across time, space and psychological typology. Additionally, cognitive psychology's significant expertise in cognitive dissection (the careful selection of task and control state which drove many cognitive neuroimaging studies in the 1980s) did not necessarily help in understanding the psychological complexities of an 'uncontrolled' state of rest. But we are now seeing the creative use in

---

[i] See Chaps. 3, 4 and 5.

cognitive neuroscience of various 'introspective' methods to attempt to capture fleeting moments of consciousness, the emergence of spontaneous thoughts and the moment of transition into a state of mind wandering.[5][ii]

In the remainder of this chapter, we consider some of the difficulties involved in characterizing the resting state in a field that has taken a particular interest in the DMN – namely psychopathology. Psychopathology researchers have increasingly adopted the DMN as a means to investigate clinical symptoms and 'atypical' internal states (see Fig. 2.1).

In part, this explosion of research results from convenience. The DMN can be identified via a resting-state fMRI scan without any task involved: a participant can simply lie in the scanner, and correlated patterns of resting brain activity – functional connectivity – can be found that highlight synchronized 'hubs' of the network. This makes it much easier to acquire data from clinical groups who may struggle with a complex task owing to problems with attention, memory or cognitive control.

Psychopathology researchers have, unsurprisingly, been interested in what the putative functions of the DMN have to tell us about particular disorders. For instance, along with introspective processes, the DMN has been linked to theory-of-mind or 'mentalizing' skills: the ways in which we understand other minds. This has led some to suggest that it may play an important role in autism spectrum disorder, which is historically characterized by problems with understanding others. For instance, an early study by Kennedy and colleagues reported that the DMN 'failed to deactivate' during standard cognitive tasks for a group of autistic adults, which they speculated could reflect 'abnormal internally directed processes at rest'.[6] Similar observations have been made in research on schizophrenia, although they have mostly been interpreted as reflecting problems with attention and memory.[7]

However, the DMN is just one of many networks that can be observed during a resting-state fMRI scan, and these other resting-state networks (RSNs) are increasingly being used to explore psychopathology. For instance, signals in sensory regions will still tend to be synchronized at rest, which allows for auditory and visual RSNs to be identified. Studying the interaction of these networks with the DMN and other brain regions at rest provides clues as to how sudden sensory experiences – such as hallucinations – can occur spontaneously from brain activity. One current idea is that hallucinations could arise from the contents of an internally

[ii] See Chap. 6.

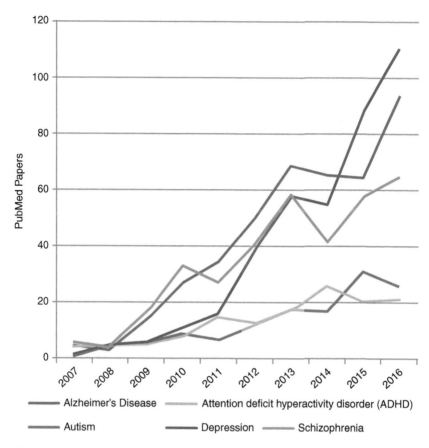

Fig. 2.1 Psychopathology papers published on 'default mode' or 'default network' (PubMed search 18 May 2016; 2016* is a projected estimate for end of year based on papers published to date)

focused state abruptly collapsing into a sensory or perceptual state if the DMN itself is unstable.[8]

Groups of regions related to cognitive control, even if usually associated with an external task rather than rest, also tend to show synchronized activity during a resting-state scan. Along with the DMN, they are also thought to interact with a third set of regions – centred around the insula and anterior cingulate – sometimes called the salience network. This network is involved in identifying significant internal and external changes that require a redirecting of attention, and has been proposed as that which controls the switch between the 'internally-focused' states of the DMN and 'externally-focused' states of other networks. This role of this network has attracted considerable interest from researchers who work on psychosis – as many psychotic experiences may seem imbued with strangely significant or meaningful qualities – and also those who research depression and attention deficit hyperactivity disorder (ADHD).

In this way, rest and the resting state have become the window through which many researchers now choose to study specific disorders. There has also arguably been a shift from researchers focusing simply on the DMN to thinking more about how various networks interact with each other over time. This is likely to be particularly important for transient states of mind such as a loss of attention, an intrusive thought or a strange perception. However, there are some important caveats around this work. One concerns methodology, and the other is an interpretative problematic.

First, resting-state scans require participants to keep still. Small head movements over time during a scan can induce systematic biases in the data, and these particularly affect the kinds of statistical analysis required to measure synchronization between brain regions. While certain methods can mitigate such problems, movement during scans has been recognized to be a significant issue, particularly for younger participants. As such, enthusiasm for early findings of connectivity alterations in the DMN in autism, for example, have had to be tempered by concern about the possible effects of participants moving around.[9]

Second, how we should interpret evidence of 'atypical' resting states remains a quandary. Research on different disorders frequently runs in parallel, with limited crosstalk. Very similar findings can therefore end up being interpreted in very different ways: one researcher's 'executive control failure' could be another's 'problem with mentalizing'. In neither case do interpretations become specific explanations.

For the DMN, this may in part reflect its origins in being a 'task-off', 'resting' state. Ever since the DMN emerged, a worry has been that the investigator does not know, ultimately, what is going on in a participant's head: the 'default mode' is a black box that allows for ever-expanding redescription and reinterpretation. When one turns to psychopathology, this problem is magnified tenfold: we know less, not more, about how to interpret the internal states of those with autism, ADHD or psychosis. And how they may differ is not necessarily mysterious: in some cases, mundane contextual factors could have a considerable effect. For example, a resting scan will often be acquired after participants have attempted other scans and tasks that are explicitly designed to measure their difficulties or impairments. This could then affect what they are thinking about at rest, in a way that differs from healthy control participants. Being aware of the individual experience of rest is crucial to avoid the possibility of atypicality in results being too rapidly interpreted as pathological.

In this respect, though research on the DMN and rest may be becoming more nuanced, the normative legacy of thinking about the DMN as driving unguided and uncontrolled processes persists in psychopathology research, as it does elsewhere. While the statement 'the resting state is not truly a resting state at all'[10] has now become a shibboleth, it remains far from clear how to parse the complex psychological processes that occur during it. While resting-state fMRI research opens up significant possibilities for understanding the dynamics of altered, unusual and debilitating states of mind, our interpretations must be tempered by a critical view of what counts as a default mode.

NOTES

1. Hans Berger, 'On the Electroencephalogram of Man: Second Report', in *Hans Berger on the Electroencephalogram of Man: The Fourteen Original Reports on the Human Electroencephalogram*, trans. Pierre Gloor (Amsterdam; New York: Elsevier Pub. Co., 1969), 84, 83. Paper originally published 1930.

2. See for example Rémi Patriat et al., 'The Effect of Resting Condition on Resting-State fMRI Reliability and Consistency: A Comparison between Resting with Eyes Open, Closed, and Fixated', *NeuroImage* 78 (2013): 463–73, in which there is explicit attention given to the effects of slightly different 'resting conditions'.

3. Marcus E. Raichle, 'The Brain's Default Mode Network', *Annual Review of Neuroscience* 38, no. 1 (2015): 434.

4. Felicity Callard and Daniel S. Margulies, 'What We Talk about When We Talk about the Default Mode Network', *Frontiers in Human Neuroscience* 8 (2014): 619.

5. For example, see Melissa Ellamil et al., 'Dynamics of Neural Recruitment Surrounding the Spontaneous Arising of Thoughts in Experienced Mindfulness Practitioners', *NeuroImage* 136 (2016): 186–96; Russell T. Hurlburt et al., 'What Goes on in the Resting-State? A Qualitative Glimpse into Resting-State Experience in the Scanner', *Frontiers in Psychology: Cognitive Science* 6 (2015): 1535.

6. Daniel P. Kennedy, Elizabeth Redcay, and Eric Courchesne, 'Failing to Deactivate: Resting Functional Abnormalities in Autism', *Proceedings of the National Academy of Sciences* 103, no. 21 (2006): 8275–80.

7. Susan Whitfield-Gabrieli and Judith M. Ford, 'Default Mode Network Activity and Connectivity in Psychopathology', *Annual Review of Clinical Psychology* 8 (2012): 49–76.
8. Renaud Jardri et al., 'The Neurodynamic Organization of Modality-Dependent Hallucinations', *Cerebral Cortex* 23, no. 5 (2013): 1108–17.
9. Ralph-Axel Müller et al., 'Underconnected, but How? A Survey of Functional Connectivity MRI Studies in Autism Spectrum Disorders', *Cerebral Cortex* 21, no. 10 (2011): 2233–43.
10. Abraham Z. Snyder and Marcus E. Raichle, 'A Brief History of the Resting State: The Washington University Perspective', *Neuroimage* 62, no. 2 (2012): 902–10.

Ben Alderson-Day is a psychologist and cognitive neuroscientist at Durham University. His work has included research on hallucination experiences in clinical and non-clinical populations, and executive function and categorization in autism spectrum disorders.

Felicity Callard is Director of Hubbub and an academic at Durham University (Department of Geography and Centre for Medical Humanities). Her interdisciplinary research focuses on the history and present of psychiatry, psychology, psychoanalysis and the neurosciences. She is co-author of *Rethinking Interdisciplinarity across the Social Sciences and Neurosciences* (Palgrave Macmillan, 2015).

CHAPTER 3

The Quest for *quies mentis*

Hilary Powell

Abstract This chapter explores the relationship between mental rest and wandering thoughts as conceived in the literature of the early medieval monastic tradition. As with contemporary neuroscientific models, medieval theologians were aware of the mind's natural propensity to roam and drift away from a task toward unrelated thoughts and feelings. While universal and unavoidable, this was nonetheless unacceptable, and monks were instructed to make every effort to still wandering thoughts. For the monks, therefore, mental rest involved unceasing vigilance and mental exertion, for it was a task which, if neglected, could lead to spiritual destitution.

Keywords Cassian · Medieval · Mind wandering · Monasticism · Quiet mind

Acquiring a still or restful mind lay at the core of the medieval Christian monastic tradition and, according to St. Anselm, the great theologian of the eleventh century, it was the goal towards which every monk ought to be oriented. In a letter written in the early 1070s, Anselm advised Lanzo,

H. Powell (✉)
Durham University, Durham, United Kingdom
e-mail: hilary.powell@durham.ac.uk

© The Author(s) 2016
F. Callard et al. (eds.), *The Restless Compendium*,
DOI 10.1007/978-3-319-45264-7_3

a novice monk at Cluny, to avoid 'a restless mind ("mentis inquietudine") … [and] devote your whole strength to attaining a "quieti mentis"'.[1] Like most medieval epistles, Anselm's letter reached a much larger audience than just Lanzo: not only read aloud to the entire Cluny community, it was also copied and circulated throughout the Benedictine order and even incorporated by his hagiographer into his saint's life.[2] The subject of restless minds ranked high on the medieval monastic agenda.

Some 900 years later, restless minds have once again garnered interest, not among theologians this time, but in the field of cognitive neuroscience. In their 2006 article entitled 'The Restless Mind', neuroscientists Jonathan Smallwood and Jonathan Schooler characterized mind wandering as 'one of the most ubiquitous and pervasive of all cognitive phenomena'.[3] The feeling of our minds drifting away from a task towards unrelated inner thoughts, fantasies and imaginings is now a feasible object of scientific enquiry. Recent neuroimaging research reveals a significant overlap between brain regions activated during episodes of mind wandering and the large-scale neural network known as the default mode network (DMN).[4] [i] Scans conducted during the so-called 'resting state', when the mind is not occupied with an explicit task, show the brain busily engaged in mental processes typical of mind wandering. In other words, the mind taking a rest from mental tasks does not rest in an idle or inert sense but remains active – roaming, wandering and inhabiting daydreams. This complex nexus of rest, unrest, mental wandering, work and attention is fascinating, and suggests an interesting lens through which we might review the medieval standpoint. Moreover, what might be the recursive effects of such an undertaking, or how might early medieval notions of mental rest and mind wandering interrogate the experimental paradigms of the cognitive sciences?

The word 'rest' derives from the Old English *ræst* (noun) or *ræstan* (verb) and is Germanic in origin, relating to a break in activity. In Latin, the closest equivalent is *requies*, 'rest from labour', which has its root in *quies*. *Quies* defies a straightforward translation since it was used as both a measure of stillness and silence. It encompassed ideas of 'rest, quiet, repose, the cessation of labour, the leading of a quiet life and keeping still'.[5] [ii] Rather than supposing the word possessed a definite meaning, we might be better off envisaging it as a concept. This is certainly how the

---

[i] See Chap. 2.
[ii] Cf. Chap. 23.

fourth- and fifth-century Christian monks living in the Egyptian desert interpreted it. A collection of sayings codifying the wisdom of the early Desert Fathers devoted an entire chapter to the subject of *quies*.[6] It was a celebrated and attractive characteristic of desert dwelling; an early visitor wrote of the desert's 'huge silence and great quiet' ('silentium ingens, quies magna').[7] Yet *quies* was also a quality or emotional state to attain, as testified by Anselm's enjoinder that a 'quieti mentis' was something to which one should devote one's whole strength. Withdrawal to the desert/monastery – the foundational principle of monasticism, known as *anchoresis* – provided the *quies* for the practice of a 'quieti mentis'.

Earlier in his letter to the novice monk Lanzo, Anselm compared monastic life to a port which offered '...shelter from the storms and tossings of the world', and cautioned him to be wary of 'disturbing the tranquility of port with the wind of fickleness and the hurricane of impatience, and [to] let his mind, lying at rest ("quieta") under the protection of constancy and forbearance, give itself up to the fear and love of God in carefulness and sweet delight'.[8] Monasticism offered a tranquil haven for the mind away from the noise of the storm and squalls of secular life. Yet despite the safe berth, the novice monk must still beware the unsettling winds of emotion that threatened his mental stillness.

In withdrawing to the desert, the early monks not only relinquished the shackles of secular life but removed themselves from all associations with their previous lives. Their goal, *theôria* in the Greek and *contemplatio* in Latin, was to attain knowledge of God, a state of grace unattainable to those still enmeshed in the vices or *passiones*. Before the monk could hope to produce the purity of prayer that would bring him close to God, a state of *apatheia*, freedom from the passions, had to be attained. John Cassian writing in the 420s gave the following advice:

> First, anxiety about fleshly matters should be completely cut off. Then, not only the concern for but in fact even the memory of affairs and business should be refused all entry whatsoever; detraction, idle speech, talkativeness, and buffoonery should also be done away with; the disturbance of anger, in particular, and of sadness should be entirely torn out; and the harmful shoot of fleshly lust and of avarice should be uprooted. (9.III.1)[9]

After the cleansing purgation, the 'unshakeable foundations of deep humility should be laid', upon which a tower of spiritual virtues 'that will penetrate the heavens' can be 'immovably fixed'. Cassian then employed an analogy, perhaps the inspiration for Anselm some 700 years later, in which he explained that the tower, 'resting on such foundations, even though the heaviest rains of the passions should beat against it like a battering ram and a savage tempest of adversary spirits should rush upon it, will not only not fall into ruin but no force of any kind will ever disturb it' (9.II.3–4). The mind, housed in its tower founded on deep humility, can withstand the destabilising threat posed by the passions.

Thus the goal of the monk was mental tranquility, to remain unperturbed or unmoved by thoughts arising from the secular world. John of Lycopolis maintained that '…through any sinful act or onset of perverse desire the devil enters into our hearts…[and] such hearts can never have peace or stillness ("quietem")'.[10] In order to eliminate one's inclination towards sinful acts, the monk submitted himself to self-abnegating or ascetic practices. Abstinence from sex, food and drink, company and conversation, clothing and even the sight of the outside world was intended to subdue bodily urges while rounds of prayer, psalmody and repetitive manual tasks such as 'basket-making' or weaving allowed the mind to meditate continuously on God. By withdrawing into oneself through such ascetic practices, the monk might achieve a state known to the Greek-speaking desert dwellers as *hesychasm* ('stillness, rest, quiet, silence') in which the monk, through unceasing wordless prayer, might receive experiential knowledge of God. St Antony, the first of the great Egyptian hermits, wrote that revelations came only to a 'calm' soul.[11] *Hesychasm*, transmitted to the Latin West as *theôria* or *contemplatio* and achievable only through a *quies mentis* ('stillness of mind'), brought a heightened relationship with God.

A mind 'at rest' or 'stilled', however, was not easily achieved. If we recall Anselm's directive, it was a task to which the monk ought to devote his 'whole strength'. Moreover, everything in his letter, he claimed, 'pertained to the preservation of a stilled mind ("ad custodiendam mentis quietem")'.[12] Stilled minds need to be maintained and defended; upkeep and observation were required. In other words, being 'at rest' took effort; it was something that a monk worked hard to achieve.[iii] Acquiring and maintaining a stilled mind was a difficult task, a fact which the Desert Fathers acknowledged. In John Cassian's *Conferences*, a set of twenty-four thematic dialogues which codified the advice he and his friend Germanus had received from monastic elders on their visit to the Egyptian desert, he returned repeatedly to the topic of restless or wandering thoughts.

[iii] Cf. Chap. 9.

He complained at the way his mind inevitably strayed during his spiritual exercises:

> My mind is infected by poetry, those silly stories of fable-tellers [like Ovid] and the tales of war in which I was steeped from the beginning of my basic studies when I was very young.... When I am singing the psalms or else begging pardon for my sins, the shameful memory of poems slip in or the image of warring heroes turns up before my eyes. Daydreaming about such images constantly mocks me and to such an extent that it prevents my mind from attaining to higher insights and cannot be driven away by daily weeping. (14.XII)

Elsewhere he spoke of 'careless and slippery digressions of thought... which prick the mind with their vague and subtle suggestiveness' (23. VII.1,5). In another *Conference*, he has Germanus describe how the mind 'wanders off in slippery streams' ('lubricus discursibus animus evagatur') and bewail the fact that even when the mind is restored to the fear of God or spiritual contemplation:

> ... before it can be fixed there, it disappears again still more swiftly. And when we apprehend, as though awakened, that it has strayed ('deviasse') from its proposed intention ... we wish to bind it with the most tenacious attentiveness of heart as though in chains, [but] in the midst of our attempts, [it] slips away, swifter than an eel from the recesses of the mind. (7.III.4)

Even when the heart is willing, it seems the mind often refuses to be stilled. But the monk should not lose hope. Cassian's complaints were met with sage advice, for although 'wandering thoughts' ('cogitationum pervagatione'), glossed as 'every thought that is not only wicked but even idle and that to some extent departs from God', were 'the most impure fornication' (14.XI.5), they were part of the human condition. In the penultimate *Conference*, Abba Theonas poses the question:

> Who can continually maintain such a fervour of spirit that he does not sometimes when slippery thoughts ('lubricis cogitationibus') take his attention away from prayer sometimes plunge from heavenly to earthly realities? ... Who has never been worried about food, clothing or concerned about welcoming brothers ... or building a cell? ... No one apart from our Lord and Saviour has so stilled ('defixa') the natural vagaries of his mind ('naturalem pervagationem mentis') and remained in constant contemplation of God

that he has never been snatched away from it and sinned for love of some earthly thing. (23.VIII.2)

In a Christian adaptation of Neoplatonist notions of the soul, the human mind in the human body cannot help but wander. Since Adam and Eve's disobedience in the Garden of Eden, wandering thoughts were an inescapable fact of life, and even monks ascending to the height of spiritual *theôria* were not impervious to wandering and restless thoughts.

If one's thoughts had to wander, the answer lay in letting them stray on to spiritual matters. This was the advice John Cassian received from Abba Nesteros: let readings and meditations upon spiritual writings replace the fables and narratives of youth, store this knowledge deep in the recesses of your mind so that 'not only every aim and meditation of your heart but also every wandering and digressive thought of yours will become a holy and continuous reflection on the divine law' (14.XIII.7). In a celebrated passage Cassian compared the human heart and mind to millstones:

> ...which the swift rush of the waters turns with a violent revolving motion. As long as the waters' force keeps them spinning they are utterly incapable of stopping their work, but it is in the power of the one who supervises to decide whether to grind wheat or barley or darnel.... In the same way the mind cannot be free from agitating thoughts during the trials of the present life, since it is spinning around in the torrents of the trials that overwhelm it from all sides. But whether these will be either refused or admitted into itself will be the result of its own zeal and diligence. For if...we constantly return to meditating on Holy Scripture,...to the desire for perfection and hope of future blessedness, it is inevitable that...the mind [will] dwell on the things that we have been meditating on. But if we are overcome by laziness and negligence and...get involved in worldly concerns and unnecessary preoccupations, the result will be as if a kind of weed has sprung up, which will impose harmful labour on our heart. (1.XVIII.1–2)

The solution to the seemingly paradoxical quest for *quies mentis*, 'a stillness of mind', lay in reading, preparing and habituating one's mind so that during its wanderings it would automatically alight on spiritual matters rather than those slippery itchings which would send the monk into sin. In short, the mind cannot be stilled but the heart need not move.

In the Christian monastic tradition, attaining a quiet mind or mental rest, a state in which the mind was no longer troubled by distracting thoughts, was a ceaseless endeavour, which required an unstinting attentiveness to the contents of consciousness. It was also unrealizable. In this respect, there is overlap with contemporary cognitive science to the extent that wandering thoughts are considered an inescapable feature of human experience: the mind is always working and whirring around. Yet where the medieval and the modern do part company is in the way rest is defined in the context of mental tasks. In the domain of the neuroscientific experiment, the 'resting state' is conceptualized as being 'off task'. Participants in neuroimaging studies of the DMN are intentionally not directed to perform mental tasks. Mental rest – the 'resting state' – is thus defined by the absence of a task. In the world of the Egyptian desert or medieval cloister, however, we find the entirely opposite view: mental rest was not only a task but one requiring sustained effort.

NOTES

1. St. Anselm, *The Letters of Saint Anselm of Canterbury*. Cistercian Studies Series, 3 Vols, ed. Walter Fröhlich, vol. I (Kalamazoo, Mich.: Cistercian Publications, 1990), 133–37.
2. Eadmer of Canterbury, *The Life of Saint Anselm, Archbishop of Canterbury*, ed. Richard William Southern (Oxford: Oxford University Press, 1962), 32–34.
3. Jonathan Smallwood and Jonathan W. Schooler, 'The Restless Mind', *Psychological Bulletin* 132, no. 6 (2006): 956.
4. Jonathan Smallwood and Jonathan W. Schooler, 'The Science of Mind Wandering: Empirically Navigating the Stream of Consciousness', *Annual Review of Psychology* 66 (2015): 487–518.
5. Charlton T. Lewis and Charles Short, *A Latin Dictionary* (Oxford: Oxford University Press, 1879).
6. 'Vitae patrum', *Patrologia Latina* 73, 858A–860C, 1849.
7. Rufinus, 'Historia monachorum in Ægypto', in *Patrologia Latina* 21, 858A–860C, 1849.
8. Eadmer of Canterbury, *The Life of Saint Anselm, Archbishop of Canterbury*, 34.
9. John Cassian, *The Conferences*. Ancient Christian Writers 57, trans. Boniface Ramsey O.P. (New York/Mahwah, N.J.: Newman Press, 1997), in text citation by conference, chapter and sub-chapter. The Latin text is printed in *Patrologia Latina* 49, 477–1328.
10. Rufinus, 'Historia monachorum in Ægypto', 396C.
11. David Brakke, *Athanasius and Asceticism* (Baltimore, Md.: Johns Hopkins University Press, 1998), 239.
12. Eadmer of Canterbury, *The Life of Saint Anselm, Archbishop of Canterbury*, 34.

FURTHER READING

Carruthers, Mary J. *The Craft of Thought: Meditation, Rhetoric, and the Making of Images*, 400–1200. Cambridge: Cambridge University Press, 1998.

Dunn, Marilyn. *The Emergence of Monasticism: From the Desert Fathers to the Early Middle Ages*. Oxford: Blackwell Publishers, 2000.

Russell, Norman, and Benedicta Ward, S.L.G. *The Lives of the Desert Fathers*. London: Cistercian Publications, 1981.

Ward, Benedicta, S.L.G. *The Desert Fathers: Sayings of the Early Christian Monks*. London: Penguin Books, 2003.

White, Carolinne. *Early Christian Lives: Life of Antony by Athanasius, Life of Paul of Thebes by Jerome, Life of Hilarion by Jerome, Life of Malchus by Jerome, Life of Martin of Tours by Sulpicius Severus, Life of Benedict by Gregory the Great*. London: Penguin Books, 1998.

Hilary Powell is a medievalist at Durham University (Department of English Studies and Centre for Medical Humanities). She is currently researching how the experience of letting one's mind wander possessed both positive and negative associations in the medieval monastic tradition.

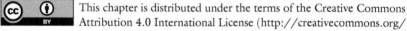

CHAPTER 4

Writing and Daydreaming

Hazel Morrison

Abstract This chapter was conceived during an interdisciplinary psychological experiment, in which geographer Hazel Morrison asked participants to record and describe in face-to-face interviews their everyday experiences of mind wandering. Questions abound concerning the legitimacy of interviewee narratives when describing subjective experience, and the limits of language in achieving 'authentic' description. These concerns increase when looking at mind-wandering experiences, because of the absence of meta-cognition during periods of self-generated thought. Here, Hazel explores the tensions at play in twentieth-century discourses around the self, fantasy and expression.

Keywords Anna Freud · Mind wandering · Psychoanalysis · Self-representation · Sigmund Freud · Virginia Woolf

The experience of mind wandering – which tends, now, to be placed by the discipline of psychology under the umbrella term 'self-generated thought', along with associated states such as daydream, fantasy and reverie – is recognized as a ubiquitous component of everyday life.[1] '[I]n day-dreaming',

H. Morrison (✉)
Durham University, Durham, United Kingdom
e-mail: hazel.morrison@durham.ac.uk

© The Author(s) 2016
F. Callard et al. (eds.), *The Restless Compendium*,
DOI 10.1007/978-3-319-45264-7_4

27

wrote Jerome Singer, 'all of us are in a sense authorities because of the very private nature of our experiences'.[2] Yet when looking to the history of psychological research that underpins contemporary understandings of mind wandering, 'all of us', that is, the generic you and I who experience our minds wandering every day, are notably absent. This isn't to say that the voices, experiences and narratives of everyday people are entirely obscured. Rather the reliability – or, one might say, the authority – of the subjective viewpoint is repeatedly denigrated.[3]

This, argue Schooler and Schreiber, is because although our experience of mind wandering is in itself undeniable, our ability to accurately represent our experience is frequently inadequate.[4] A momentary loss of 'meta-cognition', or self-reflexive awareness of our mental state, is commonly recognized to characterize the transition to the mind wandering state.[5] And if we are unable to recognize our minds having wandered, the validity of our accounts of these fugitive mental processes must be questionable. There are historical precedents to this problematic. The psychologist William James, for example, famously compared the attempt to capture such fleeting subjectivity as that of grasping 'a spinning top to catch its motion, or trying to turn up the gas quickly enough to see how the darkness looks'.[6]

I agree that the aforementioned denigration of the authority of subjective experience may be traced to this long-standing issue of meta-cognition, and its absence during periods of mind wandering. However, James recognized a second impediment to introspection, which, until recently, has received little attention within mainstream psychology. This he identified as the limitation of language, claiming an 'absence of a special vocabulary for subjective facts', which hindered the study of all 'but the very coarsest of them'.[7] More than a century on, Callard, Smallwood and Margulies, in a commentary on scientific investigations of the mind at 'rest', recognize a similar problematic. A 'historical bias', they write, 'toward explicating external processing has meant the psychological vocabulary for describing internally generated mental content is relatively stunted.'[8] Nonetheless, they suggest there exist pockets of literature, now 'largely unknown or disregarded in cognitive psychology' which once used heterogeneous methods to study and elicit states of 'daydream, fantasy, mind wandering and dissociation'.[9]

To bring some of these methods to greater visibility, this chapter looks back to the period 1908–23, a period during which daydream and fantasy were experimentally explored through diverse introspective practices, ranging from the free association methods of psychoanalysis to stream of consciousness literary techniques. Reading Sigmund Freud's famous essay 'Creative Writers and Day-Dreaming' (1908), in relation both to his daughter Anna Freud's essay 'The Relation of Beating-Phantasies to a Day-Dream' (1923) and to Virginia Woolf's short story 'The Mark on the Wall' (1919), this chapter explores the place of writing within complexes of daydream and fantasy. These interconnected texts make clear the complexities of articulating inner, mental phenomena through the medium of the written word. In so doing, they offer additional paths through which we might understand why the subjective viewpoint has often been denigrated or downplayed within the history of daydreaming and mind wandering research.[i]

MULTIPLICITY OF THE SELF AND THE FRAGILITY OF SELF-REPRESENTATION

Sigmund Freud's essay 'Creative Writers and Day-Dreaming' (1908) is known for its long-standing contribution to studies of daydream and fantasy, phenomena now frequently brought into confluence with mind wandering.[10] Freud recognized imaginative activities such as daydreaming, 'phantasy' and building 'castles in the air' as normal human behaviour. Yet despite the ubiquitous nature of daydreaming, he understood it to necessitate concealment.[11]

Why? Freud identified socially unacceptable egoistic and erotic wishes as significant motive forces that furnish the contents of fantasy and daydream. Freud wrote of the 'well-brought-up young woman' being 'allowed a minimum of erotic desire', and of the young man who must learn to subdue an 'excess of self-regard' to gain acceptance in society. At the extreme, to allow one's daydreams to become 'over-luxuriant' and overpowerful was seen to risk the onset of 'neurosis or psychosis'.[12]

Only the creative writer, argued Freud, was uniquely able to articulate 'his [sic] personal daydreams without self-reproach or shame'. The aesthetic qualities of prose were seen by Freud to 'soften', 'disguise' and sublimate the egotistical elements of the daydream, allowing author and reader alike covert indulgence in the pleasure of fantasizing.[13] [ii]

---

[i] See Chap. 5.
[ii] Cf. Chap. 7.

CREATIVITY, SELF AND SUBLIMATION:
'THE MARK ON THE WALL'

Virginia Woolf's short story 'The Mark on the Wall' (1919) exemplifies the skill of the creative writer in giving expression to daydream, reverie and fantasy. Like Freud, Woolf recognizes the commonality of the experience of daydreaming: even the most 'modest mouse-coloured people', claims the narrator, cherish moments of self-referential imaginative indulgence, despite believing 'genuinely that they dislike to hear their own praises.'[14] Moreover, Woolf's text addresses how, for daydream and fantasy to be freely expressed, the writer must deploy tactics of disguise and deflection.

Woolf's experimental approach to depicting inner monologue mimics the rhythms and effects of the wandering mind, as her writing gravitates from domestic space towards thoughts of childhood fancy. The sight of burning coals evokes description of a 'calvacade of red knights ... an old fancy, an automatic fancy, made as a child perhaps'. Distracted, her thoughts 'swarm upon a new object': a poorly perceived mark, 'black upon the white wall ...'. Rich and humorous, her prose flits from some current impression (a bowl, flower, cigarette smoke) to self-referential thoughts and fantasies. Intermittently her train of thought returns to the mark on the wall: lifting this new object up 'as ants carry a blade of straw so feverishly', before leaving it to be picked up later, afresh.[15]

While Woolf's text meanders, and on occasion tumbles, from one thought to the next, a succession of passages offers the opportunity to reflect on the thought processes that permit fantasized, egotistical self-expression. 'I wish I could hit upon a pleasant track of thought', states the narrator, 'a track indirectly reflecting credit upon myself'. These, she continues, 'are not thoughts directly praising oneself'. Rather, they express indirectly a figure of self, 'lovingly, stealthily ... not openly adoring'. This, declares Woolf's narrator, 'is the beauty of them'.[16]

Woolf portrays daydreaming as a mode of thought that allows for the creation of a sense of self invested with depth, colour and romance. Yet the author also recognizes an inherent danger in giving voice to daydream and fantasy. Woolf's text hints at deep motivations for concealment and sublimation, for like Freud, she writes of the urge to protect the idealized self-image from the gaze of the external world. If this idealized self-image were to be openly recognized, its integrity would become threatened. To have one's fantasized sense-of-self disappear is, for the narrator, to become 'only a shell of a person', as seen by others. Indeed, writes Woolf, 'what an airless, shallow, bald, prominent world it becomes!'[17]

For the protagonist of the story, the destruction of an inner self-image that exists within the realm of fantasy is a genuine threat. Fear lies with the potential for 'idolatry', for a sense of self being 'made ridiculous, or too unlike the original to be believed in any longer'. In this sense, Woolf's short story suggests why daydream, fantasy and mind wandering are states of mind that resist introspective redescription: to give self-expression to the wandering mind is to risk damaging the inner self. Writing, I suggest, emerges as a crucial intermediary for Woolf, through which the fantasized self may be given self-expression.[18]

FRAGMENTATION

[I]n the daydream each new addition or repetition of a separate scene afford[s] anew opportunity for pleasurable instinctual gratification. In the written story ... the direct pleasure gain is abandoned.[19]

Anna Freud – as the quotation above from her essay 'The Relation of Beating-Phantasies to a Day-Dream' (1923) indicates – offers another model for the complex relationship between daydreaming, subjectivity and writing. In this essay, she presents the case of a young female patient, characterized by a strong propensity to daydream. The girl, Anna Freud writes, had a history of fantasy thinking in which two polarized thought patterns dominated. By encouraging the girl, during analysis, to express the contents of these daydreams, Anna Freud explores how processes of repression and transformation link the inner daydream to its articulation in the 'real' world.[20] In doing so, she postulates more precisely than Sigmund Freud *how* daydreaming experience is transformed and transfigured once communicated through the written word.

In Anna Freud's essay, the girl's early fantasies of beating are shown to have culminated in masturbatory climax. As the girl aged, these fantasies were increasingly repressed as the girl associated them with shame and displeasure. The girl was then reported to have developed seemingly converse daydreams, which she labelled 'nice stories'. These are understood by Anna Freud as the transformation of the beating fantasy into stories acceptable to the girl's sense of morality, which yet enable a similar degree of pleasurable gratification.

In both the beating fantasies and 'nice' daydreams, Freud relates that the girl 'did not feel bound to work out a logical sequence of events' of the kind that would characterize a written narrative. Rather she scanned forward and back to differing phases of the tale; she might 'interpose a new situation between two already completed and contemporaneous scenes', to the extent that the 'frame of her stories was in danger of being shattered'.[21] Each repetition and addition to the daydream was understood to enable renewed opportunity for 'pleasurable instinctual gratification'. Yet when the daydream became 'especially obtrusive', the girl turned to writing, reportedly 'as a defence against excessive preoccupation with it'.[22]

Anna Freud noted a sharp difference between the unbridled, multi-layered sequence of events that made up the daydream, and the structured, novelistic quality of daydreams transformed into a written story.[iii] No longer a series of overlaid, repetitive episodes, culminating time and again in pleasurable climax, once written down the 'finished story' reportedly did 'not elicit any such excitement' as during the experiencing of the daydream. Yet this, concluded Anna Freud, put her patient 'on the road that leads from her fantasy life back to reality'.[23] Like Sigmund Freud, who wrote that even if an individual were to communicate his or her phantasies they would leave the listener cold, Anna Freud recognized the role of language in transforming the affects that accompany the daydream. Outside the psychoanalytic encounter, fantasy thoughts are placed within a more linear, textual framework that flattens the dynamic nature of such thinking.[iv]

Taking these three texts together, we might relate the suspicion of everyday introspective accounts of mind wandering at least in part to the complex relations tying daydream and fantasy to the written word. Language, embedded within distinct social contexts, is in many ways considered duplicitous in relation to the contents of consciousness. Even if literary techniques, such as Woolf's, attempt to evoke the rhythms and affects characteristic of the wandering mind, writing itself is the site of an opacity that accompanies the unfurling of inner life into the social world. As James noted more than a century ago, the '*lack* of a word' imposes limitations on language's ability to represent inner experience, complicating any straightforward relationship between experience and expression.[24]

[iii] Cf. Chap. 10.
[iv] Cf. Chap. 6.

Acknowledgements This work was supported by the Volkswagen Foundation.

NOTES

1. Jonathan Smallwood and Jonathan W. Schooler, 'The Restless Mind', *Psychological Bulletin* 132, no. 6 (2006): 947.
2. Jerome L. Singer, *The Inner World of Daydreaming* (New York: Harper, 1966), 6.
3. See also Anthony Jack and Andreas Roepstorff, 'Introspection and Cognitive Brain Mapping: From Stimulus-Response to Script-Report', *Trends in Cognitive Sciences* 6, no. 8 (2002): 333–39; Felicity Callard, Jonathan Smallwood, and Daniel S. Margulies, 'Default Positions: How Neuroscience's Historical Legacy Has Hampered Investigation of the Resting Mind', *Frontiers in Psychology* 3 (2012): 321.
4. Jonathan Schooler and Charles A. Schreiber, 'Experience, Meta-Consciousness, and the Paradox of Introspection', *Journal of Consciousness Studies* 11, no. 7–8 (2004): 17–18.
5. Jerome L. Singer, 'Daydreaming, Consciousness, and Self-Representations: Empirical Approaches to Theories of William James and Sigmund Freud', *Journal of Applied Psychoanalytic Studies*, 5, no. 4 (2003), 464.
6. William James, *The Principles of Psychology*. Vol. 1 (New York: Dover, 1950), 244.
7. Ibid., 195.
8. Callard, Smallwood, and Margulies, 'Default Positions', 3.
9. Ibid.
10. Sigmund Freud, 'Creative Writers and Day-Dreaming' (1908), in *The Standard Edition of the Complete Psychological Works of Sigmund Freud*, trans. and ed. James Strachey (London: Hogarth Press: The Institute of Psycho-Analysis, 1953–74), 9: 144–45.
11. Ibid., 144–5.
12. Ibid., 146–7.
13. Ibid., 152.
14. Virginia Woolf, *The Mark on the Wall* (Richmond, Surrey: Hogarth Press, 1919), 4.
15. Ibid., 1.
16. Ibid., 5.
17. Ibid.
18. Ibid.
19. Anna Freud, 'The Relation of Beating-Phantasies to a Day-Dream Freud' (1923), in *Introduction to Psychoanalysis: Lectures for Child Analysts and Teachers, 1922–1935* (London: Hogarth Press and The Institute of Psycho-Analysis, 1974), 154–5.
20. Ibid., 157.

21. Ibid., 146.
22. Ibid., 154–5.
23. Ibid., 157.
24. James, *The Principles of Psychology*. Vol. 1, 195–6.

FURTHER READING

Callard, Felicity, Jonathan Smallwood, Johannes Golchert, and Daniel S. Margulies. 'The Era of the Wandering Mind? Twenty-First Century Research on Self-Generated Mental Activity'. *Frontiers in Psychology: Perception Science* 4 (2013): 891.
Corballis, Michael C. *The Wandering Mind: What the Brain Does When You're Not Looking*. Chicago: Chicago University Press, 2015.
Freud, Sigmund. *The Interpretation of Dreams*. Translated by Joyce Crick. Oxford: Oxford University Press, 1999.
Schooler, Jonathan W., Jonathan Smallwood, Kalina Christoff, Todd C. Handy, Erik D. Reichle and Michael A. Sayette. 'Meta-Awareness, Perceptual Decoupling and the Wandering Mind'. *Trends in Cognitive Sciences* 15. no. 7 (2011): 319–26.
Woolf, Virginia *To the Lighthouse*. Edited by David Bradshaw. Oxford: Oxford University Press, 2006.

CHAPTER 5

Daydream Archive

Felicity Callard

Abstract Felicity Callard's interest in the long history of research into daydreaming, fantasy and reverie, and the ways in which this subterranean tradition might productively complicate contemporary cognitive scientific investigations of mind wandering, has been a significant focus of her work for Hubbub. In this chapter, she conjures up an imaginary archive of the daydream, as yet dispersed across disciplinary fields and points in time and space, alludes to some of its heterogeneous contents, and asks what the power of such an archive-to-come might be.

Keywords Digression · Fantasy · History of psychology · History of the human sciences · Mind wandering

'People would rather be electrically shocked than left alone with their thoughts.' Such was the title that *Science* used to report on a study in which college students, left in a room with only their own company, seemed to prefer 'doing mundane external activities' and even to 'administer electric shocks to themselves' rather than be left with their own thoughts. The

F. Callard (✉)
Durham University, Durham, United Kingdom
e-mail: felicity.callard@durham.ac.uk

© The Author(s) 2016
F. Callard et al. (eds.), *The Restless Compendium*,
DOI 10.1007/978-3-319-45264-7_5

35

researchers ended their article with the strong – and disputable – claim: 'The untutored mind does not like to be alone with itself'.[1] Their study is one of many recent scientific contributions to a bulky and heterogeneous body of work (which extends across many centuries,[i] and involves many kinds of practitioners) that both investigates and makes strong interpretations about the shape, qualities and content of humans' inner worlds when they are not predominantly attending to the world outside. The terms used are many: daydreaming, mind wandering, fantasy, wool-gathering, stimulus independent thought, reverie. The extent to which they could be said to describe the same phenomenon is open to debate, and indeed to historically nuanced contestation. The complexity and opacity of such experiences – how difficult they are to relate to ourselves let alone to others, how closely they seem bound to our very experience of being human – seems not to dent the desire of many both to generalize and to make judgments about them. (Another recent exemplar is the psychological study titled 'A wandering mind is an unhappy mind'.)[2]

I am interested in how investigations and interpretations of daydreaming and associated states (mind wandering, fantasy and so on) variously construe particular kinds of inner experience as estimable, pathological, normative, dangerous or constitutive of particular kinds of subjectivity. They reveal a great deal about the assumptions we all make, whether we are scientists or not, about the wandering mind – its ability to open up and fold away the self; the strange temporal and spatial logics that are constituted through its wandering; its capacities both to shield its owner from, as well as render her vulnerable to, the world beyond her head; its ability both to separate itself from, and yoke itself to, the peregrinations of the body; and its potential to enjoin other minds to trace new political and social worlds. Various accounts of the daydream, or of the wandering mind, open different possibilities for understanding how the world gets inside us, and for how our inner life can feel, at times, as though it colonizes the world. When does the daydream tip into the hallucination? How has its border with the night dream experienced its own conceptual wandering, across different times and in different locations? And which kinds of settings and environments have been privileged in deliberate attempts to elicit – whether in others, or in ourselves – the daydream? For it is not only when physically alone that we can be alone with our thoughts. How, then, does the daydream take up habitation when its host is in the

<hr>

[i] See Chaps. 3 and 4.

company of others – and what are the methods that others have used in attempting to spot that move?[3]

If Jerome Singer, one of the architects of twentieth-century scientific research on these topics, is correct to describe daydreaming as 'so elusive a phenomenon',[4] that does not gainsay the fact that the daydream, in – *and perhaps because of* – its very elusiveness, calls for its own archive. The historian of science Rebecca Lemov writes of the efforts, at times overweening, that were made by human scientists after the Second World War to record the dreams, stories and intimate thoughts of a vast number of people across the world (many of them colonial subjects). She exposes a powerful desire on the part of these researchers to 'collect traces of subjectivity itself, to make an archive of the inner contents of the mind'.[5] Those human scientists are not alone in their efforts to pinion and to anatomize the shifting shapes of the moving mind.

From what, then, might the archive of the daydream be built? It would contain carefully planned attempts to elicit, capture, represent and store the daydream. It would contain the ghosts of different kinds of experimental apparatus, used in different kinds of settings. It would include the graphical marks of creative writers, traces of scientists engaging in reverie as part of their experimental procedures[6] and photographs of research psychologists' laboratories. It would contain the scales and measures that have been developed in the hope that their mesh would help disaggregate the elements of the daydream.[7] It would include case histories documenting daydreams that were unravelled in psychoanalytic consulting rooms. It would build on archival repositories that have attempted systematically to preserve the fugacious alongside the durable.[8] But it would also contain records of daydreams that have erupted even when not actively sought out or elicited: the many school records that have lamented a pupil's tendency to be lured away into a fantasmatic world beyond the classroom, alongside recent case reports in clinical literatures that mark the emergence of the new category: 'excessive' or 'maladaptive' daydreaming.[9]

This archive would also be constituted from writings that harness daydreaming and mind wandering to make adjudications about different kinds of people. '[R]everie is the automatic mental action of the poet', wrote nineteenth-century physiologist William Carpenter: the poet, unlike the 'reasoner' with his [sic] commitment to abstraction, 'give[s] the reins to his Imagination, whilst gazing fixedly upon some picturesque cloud, or upon the every-varying surface of a pebbly brook' – leaving his 'thoughts and feelings' to wander 'hither and thither'.[10] Carpenter is one of many in his efforts to install distinctions between human 'types' by dint of their resort to daydreaming, or for their tendency to daydream in different ways and about different kinds of things. A proclivity to daydream has, for example, on a number of occasions in the twentieth century been tightly tied to adolescence, as well as regarded as early evidence of psychosis in children.[11] It has been, and remains till today, a common mark of psychopathology. This putative archive would also take an interest in who has held, at different historical moments, the authority and the power to elicit, collect and anatomize the tangled workings of others' mental wanderings. We might also consider how that archive would grow if we started from the position that the daydream is constituted through and as a *collectivity* rather than hiding in the depths of one lone mind.[12]

RUMMAGING THROUGH THE ARCHIVE

I am in the midst of rummaging through fragments that I believe would belong to the archive of the daydream. I am focusing on experimental investigations that took place across what we could call the long twentieth century. These stretch from the heterogeneous efforts made by psychologists, psychoanalysts, psychiatrists and neurologists in the fin-de-siècle to delineate and track fantasies, reverie and daydreams, up to the recent efflorescence of cognitive neuroscientific research on mind wandering, which has accompanied the rise of resting-state functional magnetic resonance imaging (fMRI) research and the focus on the brain's default mode network.[ii] Research on wandering and daydreaming has, after several decades of being marginalized in psychological research, come in from the cold. The terrain of the daydream has today been claimed, in terms of scientific approaches, by cognitive psychological models. (These include the hypothesis of the decoupling of attention and perception so as to allow the brain efficiently and adaptively to process streams of external and internal information.)[13] The number of publications and experiments on mind wandering within cognitive neuroscience today implies that the dispersed archive of the daydream is growing prodigiously.

In rummaging through older parts of this would-be archive – in tracing the subterranean histories and geographies of the daydream – I

[ii] See Chap. 2.

wish not only to contribute to the historical geography of the human sciences. I want, too, to think through how such histories might be used to put pressure on today's psychological models of mind wandering. There is, I believe, the possibility of cross-pollinating, or even infecting, current scientific models with older accounts of the daydream, fantasy or reverie. The daydream archive holds multiple maps for how to navigate the putting together of bodies, minds and settings: rather than being read as historical artefacts, those maps might have utility for mind wandering wayfarers today.

If I have called my method one of rummaging, it is also one of daydreaming. I am moving across different disciplinary terrains, and encountering along the way different practices and methods of observation and elicitation for capturing the daydream, the fantasy and the travels of the wandering mind. This I experience, often, as a barely structured journey, one that feels its way and is alive to the pleasures of digression.[iii] Those different practices and experiments throw up models of the mind, and of the external and internal world, that are often incommensurable with one another. But, like the images and elements of a daydream, they can sit, somehow, cheek by jowl, rather than push one another out.

Such divagation through the archive of the daydream, then, might serve to throw up other ways of narrating the history of today's scientific field of mind wandering research – as well as displace some of the preoccupations of the present. Today's mind wandering models have emerged in the shadow of cognitive psychological task-based analyses. And these bring with them the frequent desire for clear distinctions that can be operationalized within experimental paradigms (e.g. 'externally focused' and 'internally focused'; focused on 'self' or 'other'; thinking of 'past' or 'future').[iv] But the work of the daydream is work that unties such distinctions. This would-be daydream archive, then, holds the traces of bodies, minds and instruments that have not adhered to clean partitions. It holds multiple elaborations of how a mind might like to be alone with itself.

Acknowledgements This work was supported both by the Wellcome Trust [103817/Z/14/Z] and the Volkswagen Foundation.

[iii] See Chap. 13.
[iv] See Chap. 6.

NOTES

1. Timothy D. Wilson et al., 'Just Think: The Challenges of the Disengaged Mind', *Science* 345, no. 6192 (2014): 75–77.
2. Matthew A. Killingsworth and Daniel T. Gilbert, 'A Wandering Mind Is an Unhappy Mind', *Science* 330, no. 6006 (2010): 932.
3. Changes in ocular motility, for example, have been used as a potential proxy for a shift into a daydreaming state; see Bonnie B. Meskin and Jerome L. Singer, 'Daydreaming, Reflective Thought, and Laterality of Eye Movements', *Journal of Personality and Social Psychology* 30, no. 1 (1974): 64–71.
4. Jerome L. Singer, *Daydreaming and Fantasy* (London: Allen and Unwin, 1976), 5.
5. Rebecca Lemov, 'Towards a Data Base of Dreams: Assembling an Archive of Elusive Materials, c. 1947–61', *History Workshop Journal* 67, no. 1 (2009), 46.
6. Tiffany Watt-Smith, 'Henry Head and the Theatre of Reverie', *19: Interdisciplinary Studies in the Long Nineteenth Century* 12 (2011). doi: http://doi.org/10.16995/ntn.595.
7. For example, the Imaginal Processes Inventory discussed in Jerome L. Singer and John S. Antrobus, 'A Factor-Analytic Study of Daydreaming and Conceptually-Related Cognitive and Personality Variables', *Perceptual and Motor Skills* 17, no. 1 (1963): 187–209.
8. In addition to the database described by Rebecca Lemov (see her *Database of Dreams: The Lost Quest to Catalog Humanity [New Haven, N.J.: Yale University Press*, 2015]), see also projects such as the Mass Observation Archive.
9. Cynthia Schupak and Jesse Rosenthal, 'Excessive Daydreaming: A Case History and Discussion of Mind Wandering and High Fantasy Proneness', *Consciousness and Cognition* 18, no. 1 (2009): 290–92.
10. William Benjamin Carpenter, *Principles of Mental Physiology: With Their Applications to the Training and Discipline of the Mind, and the Study of Its Morbid Conditions*, 6th ed. (London: Kegan Paul, Trench & Co., 1888), 544, 545.
11. Stanley Hall, in his monograph on adolescence, argued that 'inner absorption and reverie is one marked characteristic of this age of transition' (*Adolescence: Its Psychology and Its Relations to Physiology, Anthropology, Sociology, Sex, Crime, Religion and Education*. (New York, N.J.: Appleton, 1904); see also Charles Bradley, 'Early Evidence of Psychoses in Children', *Journal of Pediatrics* 30, no. 5 (1947): 529–40.
12. Ernst Bloch, *The Principle of Hope*, trans. Neville Plaice, Stephen Plaice, and Paul Knight, Vol. 1 (Cambridge, Mass.: MIT Press, 1995).
13. Jonathan Smallwood and Jonathan W. Schooler, 'The Science of Mind Wandering: Empirically Navigating the Stream of Consciousness', *Annual Review of Psychology* 66 (2015): 487–518.

FURTHER READING

Crary, Jonathan. *Suspensions of Perception: Attention, Spectacle, and Modern Culture.* Cambridge, Mass.: MIT Press, 1999.

Lofgren, Orvar, and Ehn, Billy. *The Secret World of Doing Nothing.* Berkeley, Calif.: University of California Press, 2010.

Felicity Callard is Director of Hubbub and an academic at Durham University (Department of Geography and Centre for Medical Humanities). Her interdisciplinary research focuses on the history and present of psychiatry, psychology, psychoanalysis and the neurosciences. She is co-author of *Rethinking Interdisciplinarity across the Social Sciences and Neurosciences* (Palgrave Macmillan, 2015).

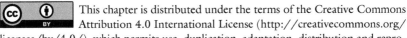

CHAPTER 6

Descriptive Experience Sampling as a Psychological Method

Charles Fernyhough and Ben Alderson-Day

Abstract This chapter outlines the practice of descriptive experience sampling (DES), a methodology with which Hubbub has experimented. Interdisciplinary DES experiments and workshops run during Hubbub's residency brought collaborators together to explore the profoundly varied ways in which the resting state can be conceptualized, and the different forms that perspectives on aspects of inner experience might take.

Keywords Descriptive experience sampling · fMRI · Inner experience · Introspection · Mind wandering · Resting state

Researchers have become increasingly interested in characterizing psychological and neural states in the absence of any specific external stimulation. It is now widely recognized that a brain that is not engaged with any particular task demonstrates highly organized patterns of activity, resonating with the much longer established idea that a 'resting' mind is anything but still. Although different terminologies have arisen to describe psychological states that are not focused on specific tasks (such as stimulus

C. Fernyhough (✉) · B. Alderson-Day
Durham University, Durham, United Kingdom
e-mail: c.p.fernyhough@durham.ac.uk; benjamin.alderson-day@durham.ac.uk

© The Author(s) 2016
F. Callard et al. (eds.), *The Restless Compendium*,
DOI 10.1007/978-3-319-45264-7_6

independent thought, daydreaming, etc.), research has cohered around the dominant term mind wandering as a designator of the varied experiences of a resting mind.[i]

Despite this growth of interest in mind wandering and the resting state, there have been few attempts to provide rich descriptions of the phenomenology (or 'what it is like' qualities) of resting cognition. One reason has been anxieties about the reliability of introspection, ranging from William James' concerns about the reliance of introspection on memory,[1] to critiques about the unreliability of participants' self-reports on the causes of their actions.[2] In attempts to avoid the methodological pitfalls of introspection, participants are typically asked, through questionnaires, to report on what was in their experience during the few minutes of the so-called 'resting-state' scan (a procedure where participants are asked to lie in the brain scanner without performing any particular task). Such catch-all reports are unlikely to provide detailed information on the complex, multi-modal and dynamic patterning of the stream of consciousness, which is likely to vary considerably in its qualities from individual to individual. Another approach has been to present participants with random probes and ask them to report on their experience at the moment of the probe. Drawbacks of that method include its likelihood of disturbing the very experiences and neural activations under investigation, and the highly constrained nature of the response options available (e.g. making a simple choice between whether one's attention was focused on the task or not). Such methodological limitations have meant that key questions about the phenomenology of resting-state cognition, such as the extent to which it has a verbal quality, remain largely unexamined.[3]

An alternative approach to characterizing a resting mind is to elicit more detailed descriptions of very specific moments of inner experience. However, extended and unguided introspective reports are open to various kinds of bias, including the effects of self-generalizations and self-theoretical attitudes. One method that acknowledges and tries to obviate such risks is descriptive experience sampling (DES). In this method, pioneered by the psychologist Russell Hurlburt of the University of Nevada, Las Vegas, the participant wears a small beeper attached to their clothing which delivers a series of random beeps to an earpiece worn in the ear. On hearing the beep, the participant's task is to make brief notes about what was in their experience in the moment

---

[i] See Chaps. 4 and 5.

just before the beep's onset. The participant then takes these notes along the next day to an in-depth interview with DES investigators, who interview the participant in great detail about the moments of experience captured in the previous day's sampling. At the heart of the method is a concern that asking people to report on their own experiences is as likely to elicit preconceptions about the nature of experience at least as much as it elicits any accurate reports on it.[ii] Crucially, DES involves an iterative method in which participants are assumed to find the task difficult at the outset and accordingly not to produce accurate descriptions. Over repeated cycles of sampling and interviewing, however, participant and investigators establish a common framework for talking about that specific participant's experiences, leading to increasing accuracy and focus of beep descriptions.[4]

Our involvement with DES research began when we started a collaboration with Hurlburt and the neuroscientist Simone Kühn at the Max Planck Institute for Human Development in Berlin. Over the course of five weeks, we trained five volunteers as DES participants, first in their natural environment (going about their daily lives in Berlin) and next in the magnetic resonance imaging (MRI) scanner. This represented the first time DES had been used in conjunction with neuroimaging.[5] Each participant underwent nine separate resting-state scans of 25 minutes each, resulting in a total of 225 minutes of resting-state functional magnetic resonance imaging (fMRI) data for each participant. In addition, each participant reported on 36 randomly sampled DES beeps collected while they were undergoing the resting-state scan. We also asked participants to complete a standard questionnaire on their experience in the resting state, the ReSQ.[6]

The results of this study have been described by Hurlburt and colleagues.[7] We found that people were generally quite consistent in what they reported in the resting state. There were considerable individual differences, for example in the reporting of inner speech, and those differences were consistent across sampling sessions. We also found considerable divergence between what people reported in DES and their responses on the ReSQ. This supports Hurlburt's contention that questionnaires generally assess participants' preconceptions about their experience at least as much as their actual experience: that is, people tend to fill in questionnaires on the basis of what they *think* their experience is like, rather than how it actually is.[iii] Although our sample size was too small to allow the drawing of firm conclusions, it was interesting that the gap between DES and ReSQ responses narrowed as participants became more expert in the sampling process.

These endeavours led to the richest body of qualitative data currently available on the phenomenology of resting-state cognition. Here are a couple of examples:

> Lara is looking at the edges of the scanner mirror – left bottom corner, and sees two of them, layering. Simultaneously she is hearing herself say, to no one in particular, 'I really want to talk to you'. The voice is recognized to be her own, expressed in her own natural way; however, the vocal characteristics are not of her own voice but of some female voice that she doesn't recognize. The wrongness of the vocal characteristics was noted only retrospectively – at the moment of the beep, experientially, Lara simply hears herself talking. She knows who the 'you' is in this sentence, but the sentence is not directed to that person. She is also seeing her hands.

> Susan innerly sees the actress Sigourney Weaver in a cryogenic tank from the movie *Alien*. She sees Sigourney's face from above, below the glass window of the tank – the rest of Sigourney's body is vaguely or blurrily present. Mostly Susan is searching for the word used in the movie: Cryogenic chamber, cryogenic tank, etc., waiting for the right word to appear. This is primarily a state of suspended animation, waiting for the word – she does not see or hear pieces of words, etc.

Our study design also allowed us to address some specific questions about the verbal nature of resting-state cognition. Covert self-directed speech (known as *inner speech*) is known to be reasonably frequent in the resting state, with one study reporting that 90 per cent of participants engaged in it.[8] In addition to classifying DES beeps according to whether they involved inner speech or not, we incorporated a standard inner speech elicitation paradigm, in which participants had to generate covert utterances in the scanner. Spontaneous and elicited inner speech related to strikingly different patterns of neural activation, casting doubt on the reliability of elicitation paradigms for this and other forms of mental experience.[9] In other words, asking people to have a particular experience in the brain scanner is no guarantee that they will do so, or at least

---

[iii] See Chap. 8.

that what results will bear much resemblance to the naturally occurring phenomenon.

One strength of DES is its capacity to describe states of experience that may be experienced by only a minority of participants – or which may even be unique to one individual.[iv] Such idiosyncratic states of consciousness are by definition very difficult to capture in self-report questionnaires. While DES studies often describe phenomena occurring in the common modalities of visual imagery, inner speech, unsymbolized thought, sensory awareness and feelings (what Hurlburt has termed the *five frequent phenomena*), the method also allows the creation of new categories if these are the best ways of describing a specific participant's experiences. For example, DES studies have shown that people's descriptions of inner speech take two forms: inner speaking and inner hearing. In inner speaking, the participant has the experience of being the producer of the speech that is experienced. In inner hearing, by contrast, the sense is more of being the recipient of the produced speech. One of our participants, Lara, showed this less common form of inner hearing, and it occurred frequently enough in her DES samples for us to compare these two forms of inner speech in a single-case design.[10]

DES is not a perfect method, and there are several grounds for caution. First, it has been argued that the act of observation inevitably changes the event itself: either in the sampling moment, or as a result of the series of interviews that follow the sampling session.[11] Second, bridging the delay between the collection of samples and the interview relies on participants being able to adequately remember enough about their experiences to report them accurately. Hurlburt has argued that variations in the time between beep and interview have made little difference to the reports he collects, as long as the delay is less than 24 hours Also important is the fact that notes on the sampled moment are taken immediately, with the iterative process aiming to ensure increasingly greater fidelity and focus of note-taking as the sampling process unfolds. However, such issues around whether observing and reporting may affect moments of experience remain a lingering concern, and one that can likely only be unpicked through further empirical research.

The various strengths and weaknesses of DES have been discussed in depth by Hurlburt elsewhere, especially with the sceptical philosopher Eric

---

[iv] See Chap. 15.

Schwitzgebel.[12] Notably, while Schwitzgebel is doubtful about the possibility of *any* kind of accurate introspection, he concludes that DES is nevertheless the most high-fidelity method for investigating inner experience currently available. Indeed, many of the criticisms levelled at DES could also be directed towards other, more superficial self-report methods: if introspection is a problem for DES, then a much larger swathe of psychological research faces similar problems.

Notwithstanding such concerns, we argue that DES represents an alternative methodology for investigating inner experience that can complement and enhance existing neuroscientific methods.[13] The richness of the data it provides also allows for current models of mind wandering and resting-state cognition to be tested against one another. One focus of our research in Hubbub has been on drawing on collaborators' expertise in mind wandering and the resting state to put such models to the test. In ongoing work, we are recoding the resting-state sampling vignettes from our Berlin study according to whether they appear to be primarily internally directed, or initiated by events in the external environment. This allows us to test a cognitive neuroscientific model of how the brain switches between internally and externally stimulated thought, opening such models up to new kinds of qualitative data.[14]

Future research will also extend the investigation into overlap between resting-state cognition and inner speech. In terms of its neural bases, inner speech activates a particular network of regions primarily in the left hemisphere of the brain. One question of interest is how language plugs in to the dynamic system that coordinates switching between on-task and task-free cognition.[15] Another focus is the idea that verbal mind wandering involves a more abstract form of inner speech, while more voluntary inner speech has a more concrete or expanded form.[16] This exemplifies one of the ways in which a focus on new kinds of qualitative data can open up novel research questions about the resting mind and brain.[v]

NOTES

1. William James, *The Principles of Psychology* (London: Macmillan, 1901).
2. Richard E. Nisbett and Timothy D. Wilson, 'Telling More than We Can Know: Verbal Reports on Mental Processes', *Psychological Review* 84, no. 3 (1977): 231–59.

[v] See Chaps. 5 and 7.

3. Ben Alderson-Day and Charles Fernyhough, 'Inner Speech: Development, Cognitive Functions, Phenomenology, and Neurobiology', *Psychological Bulletin* 141, no. 5 (2015): 931–65.

4. Charles Fernyhough, *The Voices Within: The History and Science of How We Talk to Ourselves* (London: Profile Books/Wellcome Collection, 2016), chap. 3.

5. Simone Kühn et al., 'Inner Experience in the Scanner: Can High Fidelity Apprehensions of Inner Experience Be Integrated with fMRI?', *Frontiers in Psychology: Cognitive Science* 5 (2014): 1393.

6. Pascal Delamillieure et al., 'The Resting State Questionnaire: An Introspective Questionnaire for Evaluation of Inner Experience during the Conscious Resting State', *Brain Research Bulletin* 81, no. 6 (2010): 565–73.

7. Russell T. Hurlburt et al., 'What Goes on in the Resting-State? A Qualitative Glimpse into Resting-State Experience in the Scanner', *Frontiers in Psychology: Cognitive Science* 6 (2015): 1535.

8. Delamillieure et al., 'The Resting State Questionnaire'.

9. Russell T. Hurlburt et al., 'Exploring the Ecological Validity of Thinking on Demand: Neural Correlates of Elicited vs. Spontaneously Occurring Inner Speech', *PLoS One* 11, no. 2 (2016): e0147932.

10. Kühn et al., 'Inner Experience in the Scanner'.

11. M. Perrone-Bertolotti et al., 'What Is That Little Voice inside My Head? Inner Speech Phenomenology, Its Role in Cognitive Performance, and Its Relation to Self-Monitoring', *Behavioural Brain Research* 261 (2014): 220–39.

12. Russell T. Hurlburt and Eric Schwitzgebel, *Describing Inner Experience?: Proponent Meets Skeptic* (Cambridge, Mass.: MIT Press, 2007).

13. Ben Alderson-Day and Charles Fernyhough, 'More than One Voice: Investigating the Phenomenological Properties of Inner Speech Requires a Variety of Methods', *Consciousness and Cognition* 24 (2014): 113–14.

14. Jonathan Smallwood, Kevin Brown, Ben Baird, Jonathan W. Schooler, 'Cooperation...' between the default mode network and the frontal-parietal network in the production of an internal train of thought', *Brain Research* 1428 (January 5, 2012): 60–70.

15. Fernyhough, *The Voices Within*.

16. Perrone-Bertolotti et al., 'What Is That Little Voice inside My Head?'; Alderson-Day and Fernyhough, 'Inner Speech'.

FURTHER READING

Smallwood, Jonathan, and Jonathan W. Schooler 'The Science of Mind Wandering: Empirically Navigating the Stream of Consciousness.' *Annual Review of Psychology* 66 (January 2015), 487–518.

Charles Fernyhough is a writer of fiction and non-fiction, and an academic at Durham University (Department of Psychology). His latest non-fiction book is *The Voices Within: The History and Science of How We Talk to Ourselves* (Profile/Wellcome Collection, 2015). He is an Associate Director of Hubbub.

Ben Alderson-Day is a psychologist and cognitive neuroscientist at Durham University. His work has included research on hallucination experiences in clinical and non-clinical populations, and executive function and categorization in autism spectrum disorders.

CHAPTER 7

The Poetics of Descriptive Experience Sampling

Holly Pester and James Wilkes

Abstract James Wilkes and Holly Pester, both poets, write here about their engagement with the descriptive experience sampling (DES) method, which stemmed from an interdisciplinary encounter with the psychologist Russell Hurlburt, and their experience of being trained as subjects in this technique. This chapter considers how DES can be used in unexpected ways to think through vexed questions in poetics about the relationship between experience and language, and the material ways in which experience might be captured. James and Holly consider the deployment of DES in the context of a poetry reading, which emerges as a space of multiple, distributed and distractable attention.

Keywords Poetry reading · Creative criticism · Experiment · Inner experience · Poetry

H.Pester (✉)
University of Essex, Colchester, United Kingdom
e-mail: hpester@essex.ac.uk

J. Wilkes
Durham University, Durham, United Kingdom
e-mail: wilkes_ja@yahoo.co.uk

© The Author(s) 2016
F. Callard et al. (eds.), *The Restless Compendium*,
DOI 10.1007/978-3-319-45264-7_7

51

Every day for three weeks we wore the earpieces in our ears and carried the gadgets in our pockets. The beep caught us out in our everyday actions (travelling, eating, cleaning, socializing, working and so on) and turned our attentions inside, into ourselves. The pause between the sound of the beep and our grabbing a pen to write the sample down was a moment of holding experience steady, ready for language.

When we were trained up in descriptive experience sampling (DES),[i] we became the subjects of a psychological experiment: subjects captured or produced by a deceptively simple assemblage of people, objects and forms of inscription. But we want to propose DES as also a poetic assemblage, an assemblage that is useful for thinking about poetry. Not for what it may or may not reveal about the common experiences of people who call themselves poets, but for the thinking it prompts about the relationships between experience, writing and speech.

Do you think I'm a fantasist? No. Do you think I'm making things up? No. Do you think I'm trying to make myself look good in front of the others? No ... Well, maybe a bit; I think you probably want your experiences to be thought *interesting*. If that's all, then what are your reservations? I guess ... I guess you seem to be running after this thing with words, and as you run after it, it flits off; or worse, as you run after it, it starts to take on the shape of the words and really *becomes* them. Do you mean that Julian Opie thing? Yeah exactly – you started off using the point-light example as an approximation, you only wanted to communicate the idea of movement conjured from fragments, but as soon as you used those words the point-light image was loose, proliferating everywhere, liable to lodge in the mind, in the hand, in the notebook,[ii] until it's hard to get back to what you really experienced. So you admit there *is* something to get back to? I'm not sure – isn't the experience elaborated in dialogue? You've used that phrase before, what do you mean by it? Elaborated? ... I mean that it comes into being somewhere in the process of speaking it. Like Heinrich von Kleist, the idea that thoughts emerge in tandem with speech? I guess so, kind of like von Kleist, though especially when the speaking happens in the presence of a zoom recorder, that silent third partner in the conversation...[iii] But yeah, I think it *is* something

---

[i] See Chap. 6.
[ii] See Chap. 13.
[iii] Cf. Chaps. 19 and 21.

Kleistian, something like a rhetorical drive, a communicative urge that pulls the experience into existence. That's like R then [*authors' note*: infant son] – when out of nothing, out of sleep, he shakes himself into a crying rage and you're bending over the cot and all your soothing tactics just feed an anguish that seems to come from nothing, from the slightest ruffle across the water. Hair trigger feedback loop, like the onset of the beep itself, which bursts like a diver pushing up towards the surface.

At the end of each interview with Russ Hurlburt we were asked, are you committed to the description of your experience? We might ask back, what does it mean to be committed to an experience? And how can the tallying description do anything but betray experience? The question a subject has to grapple with really is: do I believe my language can communicate interior experience, or in the attempt will I slide off the path into what Denise Riley calls linguistic unease? How invested am I in the kind of significance I have given the captured experience just by framing it in speech? In the interview we elaborate on notes scribbled down at the moment we hear the beep. These spoken accounts and their transcriptions of the experience are therefore what becomes the evidence of the experience.

This act of *elaboration*, working out (*ex* + *laborare*) through language is a work of transforming crude materials into something crafted. As the act of elaboration takes place, matter is developed into a product through the heightened application of a medium, in this case speech. A narrative is sculpted into shape, and the shape becomes data. Therefore this is not just a question of description but also of an eccentric performance of the data. Or perhaps it's true to

Elaboration: a process of working out. The interview isn't about representing a pre-given experience but about building it into being. In specialized usage, according to the dictionary, elaboration is 'the changes undergone by alimentary substances from their reception into the body to their complete assimilation'. A way of digesting experiences and transforming them into a tissue. A tissue of what? Of sound, woven between the two poles of the dialogue. Elizabeth Wilson writes about our first mind being a 'stomach-mind'. She draws on Melanie Klein to understand the primordial biological and visceral experience – the empty or full stomach of the newborn child – as also a realm of phantasy, of the psychic. If I was talking raw and cooked, about the crude materials of experience becoming language

say that through elabora-
tion the sample descrip-
tion becomes eccentric to
the experience. Through
elaboration the expe-
rience becomes imper-
sonal: I write it up and
then I speak it. I go to
speak directly from the
notes but I start to speak
from a memory as well.

OR:

in the interview, that would clearly be a
flawed description (experience itself being
shot through with the linguistic). But if we
follow Wilson – and many other feminist
thinkers – in understanding all objects to be
alloyed, entangled or impure, then we don't
need to be bound to the idea that this kind
of digestion involves a definitive change of
state (from phenomenal to linguistic, from
apprehensible to communicable). We're less
used to thinking of digestion as a communal,
shared activity – but that's what I want to
think about now.

Ruminants' teeth move side to side, helping to grind fibrous plant
matter down before it reaches their obscenely numerous stomachs. This
half-remembered fact from the biology classroom prompts me to wiggle
my own jaw back and forth. There's a flexibility here that the pure car-
nivore, with its straight meat-slicer action, lacks. That back and forth is
key to the ruminatory, digestive activity that the interview performs and
inscribes. Back and forth between interviewer and interviewee, but also
between contradictory statements, between affirmation and self-correction,
between slippages of time that are often unresolvable. This kind of communal digestion is inherently relational: it matters who you eat with because
their peristaltic actions, their digestive juices as well as yours are enacting
this transformation, this destruction and reconstitution. What it produces
must be mutually assimilable, must be something you can both swallow,
and if it isn't you'll have to chew it over until it is.

I think about the act of writing and how this makes the experience less
personal. And then I wonder if the experience ever was personal. In this
experiment the word 'experience' becomes an emblematic term for throw-
away, randomly isolated phenomena: sensations and thoughts heard and
spoken to ourselves, events imagined and fantasized. It refers to whatever
is caught in the tiny frame of the beep, rather than to experience as the
broader, ongoing agitations of inner self.

The material capture of this kind of experience, through the assemblage of beeper, subject, scrap of notepaper and interview, is more about
what lends itself to script, to being inscribed, than it is about the self. The
little moment of the beep and its description is like a process of composition. The beep isolates a feeling, removing it from the continuum of inner

communication, and transforms it into an object to be elaborated on in various media. As with the composition of an image or phrase in photography or poetry, 'experience' is formed into a distinct object with its own material support.

DES is founded on a pragmatic supposition about language. That we might exchange words as tokens for things, that we might trade them and by doing so get closer and closer to the thing itself. That there is such a 'thing itself' uninflected by how we choose to name it or the linguistic angle we approach it from. Poetry, on the other hand, comes at this from almost the opposite direction: it's deeply invested in the ability of language to invent the world. Or, if that sounds too grandiose, the ability of language to create viable paracosms, alternate realities that might *stand against* the dominant one. Many artistic forms do this, but none of them uses language in quite such a thickened way as poetry does. Its linguistic surface is a treacherous one, full of unexpected temporal loops, rhythms and sounds, which rock ambivalently underfoot, sudden blind corners inserted into the long corridors of language.

When a book is in front of us we can pick our way through this field, stopping to consider particular linguistic outcroppings or roll them in our mouths, pausing to unknot something half understood, flicking back to a line we remember or misremember. But the poetry reading, that strange scene where the poet stands before us to read their work, even if they were no more than its brief and narrow conduit, often vibrating with nervousness – this scene forbids the readerly kind of back and forth, and institutes instead a different set of relations. We think the basis of these relations is a kind of suspended attention which enables a *travelling with* the poem, and allows you to be at some distance from it at any given time, though always with the possibility of being plunged back into it.

A beep went off when I was at a poetry reading. The experience I recorded was very precise and easily accountable: at the moment of the beep I was feeling a tightening in my throat upon hearing the poet utter the words Margaret Thatcher. The sequence of events occurred over a fraction of a second: the poet said that name, my throat tightened ('like the pain of crying', I said in my interview) and then the beep went off. The clarity of this inner experience created a strange reversal of focus. My exterior life that centred me in the room and in the world receded, and interior life, the tautening inside of my neck, quickened into a retrievable thing.

This 'sample' brought to my awareness something about the experience of listening to poetry, specifically about the material effects of words. I always intuited that having poetry read to you, and being subjected to the elaborated lexicons and sounds, provoked a mix of felt and thought responses. But this little event made evident the actuality of words and their violence on the body, the fact that words and phrases can incite physical reaction.[iv]

We set up a poetry reading at which the audience were beeped through speakers at four points in the proceedings. The audience members were asked to note down their inner experience at the points of the beeps that interrupted the poetry. We looked at the samples later that day and compared them, trying to see if there was a common experience of the event.

The interviews with three trained subjects showed an intense heterogeneity of experience: a close focus on particular sounds and their delivery, a generalized awareness of background hisses, florid fantasies that a poet was speaking through a hole in their shoe, and recalled voices from earlier in the day which ventriloquized words relating to the text. Of course the experiences were different; people are different. But I think it also has something to do with the way poetic language both holds and releases attention. Under its influence, the time and space of the reading can become a halo or else an atmosphere of experience, a loosely coherent object created by the common will of a group of people agreeing to gather with intention around words spoken aloud, something which allows a common travelling, variously spiked and temporally smeared.

At a poetry reading, a communicative force is passing between and across the group, and communication of any kind, within a single person or any group, transgresses the limits of individuation. The DES interview begs me to return the experience back to individuation, through the creation of a personalized narrative,[v] and more so since this narrative is treated as something over which contracted ownership is possible. However, the more I write it and speak it the more impersonal it becomes. Therefore, experience devolves into data, into property. But the beep reminds me of the post-human notion that the subject is always immersed in and immanent to a network of relations that bridge the human and non-human. While the beep sounds the myth of personal, human, individual experience, it's more truly signalling my communicative relation to objects (like the gadgets in my pocket) and viral, animal connection to the bodies around me.

AND:

[iv] See Chap. 16.
[v] Cf. Chap. 4.

FURTHER READING

Braidotti, Rosi. *Metamorphoses: Towards a Materialist Theory of Becoming.* Cambridge, UK and Malden, Mass.: Polity Press in association with Blackwell Publishers, 2002.
Deleuze, Gilles. *Dialogues.* Translated by Claire Parnet. New York, N.Y.: Columbia University Press, 1987.
von Kleist, Heinrich. 'On the Gradual Production of Thoughts Whilst Speaking'. In *Selected Writings,* edited by David Constantine, 405–409. London: J. M. Dent, 1997.
Riley, Denise. *The Words of Selves: Identification, Solidarity, Irony.* Stanford, Calif. Stanford University Press, 2000.
Wilson, Elizabeth A. *Gut Feminism.* Durham, N.C.: Duke University Press, 2015.

Holly Pester is a poet working in experimental forms, sound and performance, and an academic at the University of Essex (in Poetry and Performance). Her work has featured at Segue (New York), dOCUMENTA 13 (Kassel), Whitechapel Gallery and the Serpentine Galleries (London).

James Wilkes is an Associate Director of Hubbub. He is a poet and writer, as well as a researcher at Durham University (Department of Geography). His interests range across contemporary and modernist poetry, audio and visual art, and their intersections with the life sciences.

CHAPTER 8

The Rest Test: Preliminary Findings from a Large-Scale International Survey on Rest

Claudia Hammond and Gemma Lewis

Abstract In this chapter, Claudia Hammond and Gemma Lewis discuss The Rest Test, the world's largest survey into people's subjective experiences of rest, devised by an interdisciplinary team at Hubbub. The Rest Test was launched in collaboration with the BBC on Radio 4's *All in the Mind*, presented by Claudia, who played a key role in the survey development. Gemma led the analysis of The Rest Test results.

Keywords BBC · Interdisciplinary · Radio · Rest Test · Subjective experience · Psychological scales

It is common to hear the complaint that in the modern world, rest is hard to find. There are too many demands on us and not enough hours in the day. Current technology leaves us permanently on call, unable to switch

C. Hammond (✉)
BBC Radio Science Unit, London, United Kingdom

G. Lewis
University College London, London, United Kingdom
e-mail: gemma.lewis@ucl.ac.uk

© The Author(s) 2016
F. Callard et al. (eds.), *The Restless Compendium*,
DOI 10.1007/978-3-319-45264-7_8

off. As we'll see later in the chapter, these perceptions might not have an entirely accurate basis in reality. Nonetheless, this is how many of us across the world feel about life today – as reflected in media headlines such as 'Stressed, tired, rushed: a portrait of the modern family'.[1]

We may complain about the incessant demands of technology such as the internet, but that same technology also provided people around the world with the opportunity to tell us what rest means to them, and gave us, as researchers, the opportunity to investigate a topic that remains empirically under-investigated. Early on in Hubbub's exploration of the topic of rest, it became clear that rest is harder to define than might be expected. A review published in 2016 emphasized that although rest is often prescribed by medical staff, the concept 'remains subjective, and is vaguely defined and often confused with sleep, limiting its utility for research and practice'.[2] But if rest is different from sleep – in that it includes conscious states – what exactly does it mean to different people? Does it refer to a rested mind or a rested body?[i] For some, the mind can't rest until the body is fully rested. For others it is the opposite: tiring out the body through vigorous exercise allows the mind to rest.

To investigate how people understand rest, Hubbub developed an online survey we named The Rest Test. In collaboration with the programmes that one of us (Claudia) presents on BBC Radio 4 and BBC World Service – *All in the Mind* and *Health Check* – we set out to recruit participants. Through appearances on TV and radio, as well as coverage in newspapers, social media and online (including a feature on whether or not people should worry about their wandering minds[3]), Hubbub reached out across the world. BBC World Service asked people to tweet pictures of how they like to rest in whichever country they live in, and listeners emailed the programmes – some writing, for example, about how difficult it is ever to feel at rest living amidst civil war.

The survey was long and required thought to complete, meaning that people had to give up 30–40 minutes of their time to fill it in. It was pointed out to us on Twitter that filling in a long survey wasn't the most restful of pursuits. However, that didn't stop people: more than 18,000 people from 134 countries attempted the survey, making this the world's largest ever survey on rest. On searching the literature, we found that previous studies investigating the concept of rest have been much smaller

[i] See also Chap. 9.

(with sample sizes ranging from 10 to 1208). They have also commonly consisted of quite selective samples, such as inpatients or nurses.[4] As the first large survey on rest administered to the general population, The Rest Test has included a broad cross section of people – anyone over 18 years old was welcome to participate.

One of our starting points was that different kinds of expertise would be necessary to design the survey. That way, we could try to ensure that our questions were broad enough to capture psychological, sociological and economic aspects of rest. During the development of the survey, Hubbub collaborators from a dozen different disciplines were consulted. After much discussion about surveys – their purpose, underpinning assumptions, and limitations – historians, social activists and sociologists began to contribute questionnaire items. Then a group of psychologists worked on the detailed construction of The Rest Test, with numerous opportunities for those from other disciplines to fine-tune questions and suggest alternatives. The resulting survey takes a somewhat unusual form. As well as the inclusion of well-validated, published scales such as the Hexaco-60[5] and the Flourishing Scale,[6] we included both specially devised questions where people could select options from long lists, and open questions to allow people to respond freely in their own words.

People completed the two-part survey online, with the option to return to the survey during the next seven days if they didn't have time to finish it. The first part covered socio-demographic data and perceptions of rest. For example, we have data on country of residence, income, gender, whether the person cared for another, levels of physical activity, benefits and disability. We also have some level of detail on people's working patterns to allow us to investigate how zero-hour contracts (which allow employers to hire staff with no guarantee of work), split shifts, worklessness and commuting times affect people's feelings about rest. If you have little choice about when to take rest, do you associate it with relaxation?[ii]

What Is Rest and How Do People like to Do It?

When we gave people a list of words and asked which word best described what rest meant to them, the most commonly cited word was relaxing, followed by peaceful/calming, comfortable, recuperative and sleep. A

[ii] See Chap. 21.

small proportion of people chose the words rare, stress-inducing, anxiety-inducing and guilt-inducing. Significantly more women than men did this. But we also gave people a free text box where they could explain in their own words what rest means to them. Table 8.1 gives a small selection of these words.

It is notable that some people selected words suggesting a more conflicted relationship with rest. The words in the right hand column indicate that rest can be hard to find or difficult to experience without feelings of guilt. Words such as 'worrying', 'challenging' and 'annoying' suggest that, for some, the negative associations with rest go even further.

We also asked people to select from a list of 25 activities those that they found most restful. Table 8.2 shows the top 20 activities. Many of the most popular activities suggest escapism, either from other people or

Table 8.1   Responses to The Rest Test question: In your own words, what does rest mean to you?

Enjoyable	Breathing space	Fields	Undisturbed	Aches
Dissociated	Clarifying	Animals	Quiet	Not permissible
Respite	Necessary	Privacy	Cooperation	Elusive
Positive	Rumination	Switching off	Peaceful	Fragile
Free	Humour	Creative	Concentration	Overlooked
Warm	Daydream	Inventive	Being dozy	Difficult to reach
Personal	Reading	Distracting	Daydreaming	Challenging
Free	Socializing	Thoughtful	Motionless	Annoying
Space	Effortlessly	Uplifting	No velocity	Worrying
Restorative	Happy	Rebalancing	Bliss	Indulgent
Fulfilling	Mindless	Laughter	Joy	Guilty secret
Quiet	Unthinking	Important	Pleasurable	Frowned upon by Others
Dreamy	Disconnected	Deliberate	Other worldly	Others
Healthy	Balance	Contemplative	Blank	Fidget
Disengagement	Energetic	Reflective	Beautiful	Selfish
Still	Not tense	Hygge[a]	Regenerative	Guilty
Healing	Enriching	Safe	Me time	Unjustified
Delicious	Sunny	Warm bath	Precious	Dark
Distracting	Sublime	Strived for	Yearned for	Waste of time
Unwind	Cool, dark	Void	Warmth	Idleness
Gift	Gentle smile	Serene	Recumbent	Feeble
Inspiring	Liberty	Recuperative	Choice	Irritating

[a]Hygge is a Danish word that is difficult to translate; 'the art of living cozily' is an approximation.

Table 8.2   Activities considered by The Rest Test respondents to be restful, in order of the most to least popular

Reading
Sleeping or napping
Looking at, or being in, a natural environment
Spending time on my own
Listening to music
Doing nothing in particular
Walking
Taking a bath or a shower
Daydreaming
Watching TV
Meditating or practising mindfulness
Spending time with animals
Spending time with friends/family
Making/drinking tea or coffee
Creative arts
Gardening
Travelling on long train journeys
Engaging in physical activity
Chatting
Drinking socially
Eating
Sexual activity
Running
Grooming
Thinking about the past

from the built environment.[iii] 'Spending time on my own' and 'being in, or looking at, a natural environment' were both ranked highly. Spending time with friends and family, and chatting and socializing came further down. When we say we need more rest, is it more that we yearn for time away from other people?

More women than men selected reading as restful, while more men selected listening to music. Notice that physical activity comes higher than chatting or drinking socially. A repeated theme in our research is that a

[iii] Cf. Chap. 12.

substantial minority considers physical exercise not to be the opposite of rest, but to be restful in itself.

The second part of the survey included several well-validated scales frequently used in psychological research. We examined well-being using The Flourishing Scale, Satisfaction with Life Scale and The Scale of Positive and Negative Experience. On this latter scale, people who said they had more rest in the last 24 hours scored more highly on subjective well-being, while people who considered themselves in need of more rest and who believe they get less rest than others scored less highly. This might suggest that rest leads to higher well-being, but we must remember that this survey takes a snapshot in time and so we can't tell which came first – the amount of rest a person believes they get or their well-being. It is possible that people who were feeling unhappy while they filled in the survey might have underestimated the amount of rest they had.

How Does the Modern World of Work Affect Our Ability to Rest?

If someone asks how things are going, many of us tend to answer, 'Oh fine, very busy. Bit too busy'. This feels true, but of course there's also an element of status in this claim. If you say you are busy, then it implies you are wanted. You are in demand. As the time-use researcher Jonathan Gershuny puts it, busyness has become 'a badge of honour'.[7] In contrast to the nineteenth century, in many parts of the world today it is work and not leisure that gives us social status.[iv]

We say we need more time to relax and that new technology means we are forever on call. But these complaints are nothing new. With each technological invention – such as the locomotive, the telephone and the telegram – people have expressed the fear that it placed more burdens upon us and made life feel more pressured.[8]

It is also common for people to overestimate the total number of hours they work. For this reason, many time-use surveys ask people to think back to the previous day or week, rather to think of a typical day or week.[9] In The Rest Test, we asked people not how much they rest in a typical day, but how many hours of rest they had in the past 24 hours. Of course, it is possible that, for some, the previous day was unusually restful or unrestful,

---

[iv] Cf. Chap. 22.

but in a large study these fluctuations should even out. When asked how much rest respondents had had in the past 24 hours, responses ranged from 0 to 14 hours, averaging at approximately 3 hours. Thirty two per cent of the people who completed the survey think they need more rest than the average person. From The Rest Test it is clear that many of us feel harried: 68 per cent would like more time to rest.

Research on time use in Europe and the United States shows that although most of us say we feel busier, average working hours have not increased in the past half century and in fact we have more spare time for resting than we used to.[10] So why doesn't it feel like that? There are several possible explanations. Time use surveys and The Rest Test provide us with averages, and so there are of course some people who have very little spare time to rest and others, who might be jobless or unwell, for example, who might have more time to rest, but who experience this as an enforced rest. Perhaps we have time to rest, but don't feel fully able to switch off, as some of those more negative words regarding rest suggest. Digital technology is often blamed here, but so far there is a lack of good evidence to suggest that screens are as bad as is sometimes claimed. Much of the time they are used to stay connected with others.

There is also another possibility, identified by the sociologist Judy Wajcman.[11] She has observed that the problem is not so much the total number of hours worked, as the irregularity of those hours. Fewer people work 9–5 than previously. How many of us could arrange on the spur of the moment to meet ten friends at 5.30 the same afternoon? Probably not very many of us, because some friends will be working, others will be picking up children or will already have other commitments. The findings of The Rest Test bear this out to some extent. People working shifts, especially shifts that include nights, considered themselves to be less rested.

The fact that thousands of people were prepared to spend time online telling us what they thought about rest demonstrates the broad spectrum of public interest in this topic. Of course, this was a self-selecting sample (and largely from the UK, the rest of Europe or North America). Perhaps the people who chose to complete the survey felt particularly strongly about the need for rest. The size of the response might also suggest that despite what we say, we like using digital technology to engage in this way. Many people, it seems, would like to have more time to rest and to have more time away from other people. Perhaps it's not the total hours resting or working that we need to consider, but the rhythms of our work, rest, and time with and without others.

Acknowledgements   The development of The Rest Test was a collaborative endeavour; contributors included Ben Alderson-Day, Josh Berson, Felicity Callard, Charles Fernyhough, Des Fitzgerald, Louise Gregor, Daniel Margulies, Giulia Poerio, Jonathan Smallwood and Tal Yarkoni.

The Rest Test was granted ethical approval by the Ethics Advisory Subcommittee, Department of Psychology, Durham University. All data from The Rest Test, together with explanations of how we analysed the data, is, at the time of writing, in preparation for submission to a peer-reviewed journal.

NOTES

1. Claire Cain Miller, 'Stressed, Tired, Rushed: A Portrait of the Modern Family' *The New York Times* (November 4, 2015), accessed June 22, 2016, http://www.nytimes.com/2015/11/05/upshot/stressed-tired-rushed-a-portrait-of-the-modern-family.html?_r=1.

2. Esther I. Bernhofer, 'Investigating the Concept of Rest for Research and Practice', *Journal of Advanced Nursing* 72, no. 5 (2016): 1012–22.

3. Claudia Hammond, 'Why We Should Stop Worrying about Our Wandering Minds', *BBC Future* (6 November 2015), accessed June 22, 2016, http://www.bbc.com/future/story/20151106-why-we-should-stop-worrying-about-our-wandering-minds.

4. See also the studies reviewed in Bernhofer, 'Investigating the Concept of Rest for Research and Practice'.

5. Michael C. Ashton, and Kibeom Lee, 'The HEXACO–60: A Short Measure of The Major Dimensions of Personality'. *Journal of Personality Assessment* 91, no. 4 (2009): 340–45.

6. Ed Diener et al., 'New Well-Being Measures: Short Scales to Assess Flourishing and Positive and Negative Feelings', *Social Indicators Research* 97, no. 2 (2009): 143–56.

7. Jonathan Gershuny, 'Busyness as the Badge of Honour for the New Superordinate Working Class. ISER Working Papers Number 2005-9' (Colchester: Institute for Social and Economic Research, University of Essex, n.d.).

8. Mark Jackson, *The Age of Stress: Science and the Search for Stability* (Oxford: Oxford University Press, 2013).

9. Liana C. Sayer, 'Trends in Women's and Men's Time Use, 1965–2012: Back to the Future? Pennsylvania State University National Symposium on Family Issues (NSFI) Book Series', in *Gender and Couple Relationships*, ed. Susan M. McHale et al. (Cham: Springer, 2016).

10. Mark Aguiar and Erik Hurst, 'Measuring Trends in Leisure: The Allocation of Time Over Five Decades', *Quarterly Journal of Economics* 122, no. 3 (2007): 969–1006.

11. Judy Wajcman, *Pressed for Time: The Acceleration of Life in Digital Capitalism* (Chicago, Ill.: Chicago University Press, 2015).

FURTHER READING

Hammond, Claudia. *Time Warped: Unlocking the Mysteries of Time Perception.* Edinburgh: Canongate, 2012.

Claudia Hammond is a broadcaster, writer and psychology lecturer. She is the presenter of *All in the Mind* and *Mind Changers* on BBC Radio 4, and *Health Check* on BBC World Service Radio and BBC World News TV. She is an Associate Director of Hubbub.

Gemma Lewis is an academic in the Division of Psychiatry at University College London. Her research currently focuses on the causes, prevention and treatment of depression using epidemiological methods and statistics.

PART II

Bodies

CHAPTER 9

From Therapeutic Relaxation to Mindfulness in the Twentieth Century

Ayesha Nathoo

Abstract This chapter is based on a talk given by historian Ayesha Nathoo at the 'Mindfulness Unpacked' symposium at Wellcome Collection in February 2016, which was linked to the 'Tibet's Secret Temple' exhibition. While the exhibition contextualized mindfulness within the Buddhist tradition, Ayesha's research on the history of therapeutic relaxation provided an opportunity to demonstrate the social and structural links between secular mindfulness and twentieth-century relaxation practices.

Keywords Muscle relaxation · Mind-body medicine · Rest · Stress · Twentieth-century history of medicine

Today's Western 'mindfulness movement' is often portrayed as a sign of and remedy for our restless, overloaded times. Contemporary mindfulness-based interventions comprise treatments for pain, mental illness and stress management and have become an integral part of preventive medicine, lifestyle and well-being agendas. In Britain, the 2015 Mindfulness All-Party Parliamentary Group report 'Mindful NationUK',[1] recommended that mindfulness be taught within schools, prisons, the workplace, and doctor and teacher training courses; there is now a burgeoning

A. Nathoo (✉)
University of Exeter, Exeter, United Kingdom
e-mail: A.Nathoo@exeter.ac.uk

© The Author(s) 2016
F. Callard et al. (eds.), *The Restless Compendium*,
DOI 10.1007/978-3-319-45264-7_9

71

industry of self-help books, audio recordings, apps and group classes on offer. As its popularity has increased, criticisms are being voiced, particularly over the individualistic, commodifiable form of 'McMindfulness', seen as complicit with a neoliberal political agenda. How have we reached this point historically and socially? And is it really all so new?

The history of mindfulness tends to be presented in one of two ways: firstly, a history that reaches back to millennia-old Buddhist teachings, from which the meditative practices and ethical frameworks derive. And secondly, a narrative starting in 1979 when the molecular biologist Jon Kabat-Zinn established what became the mindfulness-based stress reduction (MBSR) programme at the University of Massachusetts Medical School, following a 'vision' he'd experienced during a *vipassanā* meditation retreat of adapting and applying Buddhist teachings to mainstream medical and popular settings. This chapter provides an alternative historical lens. It demonstrates how Western, secular, mindfulness-based interventions both structurally and culturally built upon teachings and understandings of therapeutic relaxation which were developed from the early decades of the twentieth century.

An oft-cited definition of mindfulness, outlined by Kabat-Zinn, is the awareness that comes from 'paying attention in a particular way: on purpose, in the present moment, and nonjudgementally'. Mindfulness practitioners often clearly demarcate relaxation from mindfulness, describing relaxation as a potential 'side-effect' of mindfulness, but not an aim in and of itself. Although relaxation may ensue, the intention is not to *try* to achieve any particular state, but rather to be open to whatever thoughts and feelings pass through the mind and body, moment by moment. My aim here is neither to reduce mindfulness to relaxation, nor to enter debates around precise definitions and comparative methodologies. Instead, I explore the ways in which the framing, proliferation and application of relaxation therapies helped to pave the way for today's form of mindfulness in the West and its widespread uptake. Nonetheless, it is relevant to note that Kabat-Zinn's original course was called the 'Stress Reduction and Relaxation Program', and relaxation terminology was embedded in his early teachings and publications before being disavowed.[2]

Overlaps between mindfulness and relaxation have changed over time, as have scientific and cultural meanings of what it means to be both 'mindful' and 'relaxed'. In the interwar years, the Chicago physician and psychologist Edmund Jacobson advocated a new and narrower definition of the term relaxation, shifting away from vernacular connotations linked to recreational pursuits. Moreover, he distinguished between the commonly linked notions of 'relaxation' and 'rest', arguing that one could be resting but tense, or active yet at ease. Jacobson developed an intricate system of 'neuro-muscular relaxation', promoted as a physiologically based, scientifically valid technique. It was designed both to prevent and treat a wide array of physical and mental conditions and enhance experiences of everyday living, if comprehensively learnt and practised. Based on the premise that it is 'impossible to be tense and relaxed at the same time', and that thought itself produced muscular tension, his technique of 'progressive muscle relaxation' was a way to alleviate both physical and emotional tension. Jacobson's method involved systematically recognizing and releasing muscular tension, in order to quieten body and mind. He also advocated 'differential relaxation', whereby only muscles essential to a particular task were used and all others were relaxed, thereby eliminating unnecessary tension. Using an instrument that could detect and display minute changes in neuro-muscular electrical activity, tension became something that could be observed, quantified and treated.

Jacobson's 1934 book, *You Must Relax: A Practical Method of Reducing the Strains of Modern Living*, outlined the myriad therapeutic applications of his system of relaxation: from nervous illness, to heart disease, insomnia and indigestion – all symptomatic of tense, overactive minds and bodies unable to keep up with the pace and demands of modern living. Jacobson considered relaxation to be far superior to the traditional remedy for many of these conditions – bed rest – given that one could remain tense when resting or even sleeping, and residual tension could serve to increase rather than decrease restlessness or 'nervousness'. Rather than a common, natural state of 'rest', muscular relaxation was a skill that needed to be taught, involving weekly instruction with a qualified physician, and one or two hours of home practice per day. Once mastered, short spells of deep relaxation could be used as a means of increasing efficiency and enjoying 'modern civilization without burning the candle at both ends'.[3][i]

Placing his method firmly in the Western, scientific, secular domain, Jacobson distanced his technique from relaxation practices and ideologies that developed in parallel, influenced by occultism and the hypnotic tradition – in particular, breathing and postural exercises taught by New Thought author Annie Payson Call, and 'autogenic training' using

[i] See Chap. 15.

visualizations, formulated by the German psychiatrist Johannes Schultz. Despite these differences, and Jacobson's exclusive focus on bodily sensations, common to all of these techniques was a belief in the connection between mind and body and the therapeutic benefits of relaxation. They also required expert teaching and disciplined practice in order to cultivate a skill and an altered relationship to modernity. Much like mindfulness today, the aim of relaxation training was not to change industrialized socio-political structures and environments, but to enable individuals to relate differently to these contexts.

Muscular relaxation was enthusiastically taken up in Britain in the 1930s, especially within the performing arts and for speech therapy. Practitioners such as speech therapist M. A. Richardson and E. J. Boome from London County Council developed classes for stammering children, and disseminated the principles and ideology of relaxation therapy to wider audiences. Their 1938 publication, *Relaxation in Everyday Life*, described how habitually practising therapeutic or 'curative' relaxation might not only help with specific ailments but profoundly change an individual's entire outlook, and by osmosis impact on wider cultures of care.[4] The authors stressed the importance and responsibility of parents, especially mothers, to learn to relax for their own health and well-being and in order to foster a better home environment for their children.[ii] Teachers and healthcare workers too were identified as professionals for 'whom the study of relaxation should be essential', in order to benefit the community at large. Over 80 years before the 'Mindful Nation UK' report, Boome and Richardson declared: 'We hope that the time will eventually come when [relaxation] will be considered an indispensable part of the training of those who are in contact with children and the sick – teachers, and nursery and hospital nurses'.[5]

Although relaxation training was applicable to all, it became especially popular amongst middle-class, child-bearing women in Britain, owing largely to the work of the obstetrician Grantly Dick-Read. In a pronatalist, eugenic socio-political context, concerned with the 'fitness' of the nation, Dick-Read sought to explain and address the relatively low birth rate among middle-class women. He suggested that their reproduction rates were being impeded by fear of the pain of childbirth. Relaxation was a means to break this fear–tension–pain cycle and enable a 'natural childbirth' (a term he coined in 1933), reduce the need for analgesics, and allow childbirth to become a positive, even spiritual experience. Although

---

[ii] See Chap. 10.

sidelined by his medical colleagues, Dick-Read gained the support of influential midwives and physiotherapists who helped design, teach and implement relaxation exercises for antenatal women. Most significantly he developed a following amongst middle-class women themselves.[6]

In 1956, Prunella Briance – a mother who had endured a traumatic still-birth of her child under conventional obstetric care – set up the still widely popular National Childbirth Trust (originally the Natural Childbirth Association), to promote the teachings of Dick-Read. Relaxation exercises in preparation for childbirth soon became a routinized part of antenatal care (Fig. 9.1).[7] In the postwar decades, antenatal teachers became leading proponents of relaxation, quick to adapt and extend teachings from the antenatal to postnatal period, both creating and meeting a demand to help mothers better manage the multiple challenges of parenthood. Meanwhile, physiotherapists extended principles of relaxation for childbirth to relaxation for pain management more generally, establishing an enduring

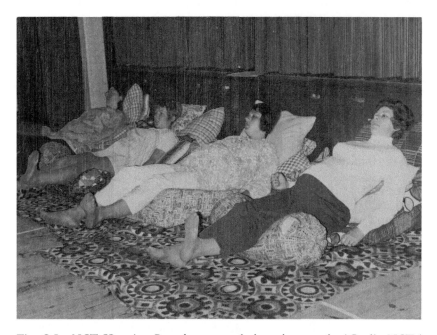

Fig. 9.1   NCT Havering Branch: antenatal class photograph. (*Credit:* NCT/ Wellcome Library, London, Wellcome Images, L0079526, released under a Creative Commons Attribution 4.0 International License (CC BY 4.0))

therapeutic role for these techniques. Relaxation became relevant for men too, especially ostensibly 'coronary-prone', overworked 'Type A' businessmen, seen as a particularly vulnerable group as physiological, psychological and epidemiological research into 'stress', 'risk-factors' and 'coping mechanisms' for heart disease developed in this period.[8]

By the 1970s group relaxation classes, as a means of 'stress management', were being offered and structured in much the same way as mindfulness classes are today. Courses involved weekly sessions guided by an 'expert' teacher, with audio recordings available for daily home practice. Course participants learnt breathing and 'deep relaxation' techniques, and were encouraged to adapt and apply 'differential' relaxation principles to everyday living. As well as relaxation instruction, classes incorporated health educational messages, group discussions, and basic scientific and physiological explanations of the body's 'fight or flight' response and the perceived detrimental impact on health and well-being of chronic exposure to stress.[iii] Relaxation was promoted as relevant and helpful for the well-being of individuals, homes, the workplace and society at large. It was framed as a safe, effective alternative to drugs for anxiety, insomnia and hypertension, and a way not only to treat ill-health, or 'dis-ease', but to encourage healthy lifestyles and boost well-being.

National and local television and radio programmes in the 1970s regularly featured relaxation discussion and teaching; and health educators, physiotherapists, general practitioners, antenatal instructors, physical education teachers, psychologists and psychotherapists all had a stake in relaxation training and promotion, and contributed to the growing self-help literature. But alongside the enthusiasm came words of caution. As one doctor signalled in a medical journal review:

> A single trip to the bookshop may well for many patients replace a series of repeat prescriptions for a benzodiazepine. Naturally however, the same caution applies to the use of relaxation as to the use of tranquillizers: one must be certain that one is not merely suppressing symptoms when it is more appropriate, if more difficult, to deal directly with an underlying cause.[9]

He also expressed concern that therapeutic relaxation instruction was aimed mainly at an 'upper-middle class audience' – the demographic who could most likely afford the training and the time to learn and effectively keep up practice. Relaxation practitioners, meanwhile, were concerned

---

[iii] Cf. Chap. 12.

about upholding the quality of teachers and demarcating 'scientific' relaxation from numerous other unregulated 'alternative therapies'. All of these issues chime with those facing mindfulness today.

Although many Western practitioners distanced therapeutic relaxation from mystical traditions, others explicitly connected it to Eastern meditative practices. One relaxation advocate explained: 'A person who learns how to relax completely – or meditate, as the Eastern teachers call it – acquires the capacity of freeing himself from fears and useless brooding over bad experiences'.[10] Yoga scholar Mark Singleton has demonstrated how yoga was reconstituted as it proliferated in the West in the postwar decades, drawing more from contemporary, Western relaxation techniques and ideologies, than ancient Indian teachings.[11] While the New Age narrative of 'Eastern wisdom' appealed to some, yoga and meditation reached far beyond the 1960s counterculture movement, and Christian as well as dharmic meditative traditions appropriated the therapeutic framework of relaxation. In the early 1970s, for example, Reverend Geoffrey Harding, head of the Churches Council for Health and Healing, founded the Relaxation Society and held lunchtime relaxation classes for city workers in his City of London church. 'By relaxing', he explained, 'we discover our own inner life, and begin to enjoy the "eternal life" that Christ was talking about. This means much more than "future life". It means Life, here and now, "Life within oneself" (St. John v. 26)'.[12]

The 1975 international bestseller, *The Relaxation Response*, by Harvard cardiologist Herbert Benson,[13] further coupled relaxation with meditation, and significantly bolstered claims of the therapeutic potential of such techniques. The book extended Benson's prior research, alongside colleague Robert Keith Wallace, into the physiological effects of transcendental meditation (TM), to include a host of 'ancient' and 'modern' methods. These included progressive muscle relaxation, yoga, meditation, autogenic training as well as repetitive prayer, all of which, Benson argued, produced similar underlying physiological changes. He defined the relaxation response as 'a physical state of deep rest that changes the physical and emotional responses to stress…and opposite of the fight or flight response'. Through lowering metabolism, blood pressure, heart rate and respiratory rate, amongst other physical indicators, Benson considered the relaxation response, however elicited, to be a powerful antidote to a whole array of stress-related conditions.

Benson significantly raised the profile of relaxation practices and 'mind-body medicine' in medical and popular arenas, no doubt helping to create a more receptive environment for Kabat-Zinn's introduction of mind-fulness into clinical settings. As Kabat-Zinn recently reflected, 'naming is very important in how things are understood and either accepted or not'. Labelling the original course the 'Stress Reduction and Relaxation Program' in 1979 was therefore a strategic choice. 'Mindfulness medi-tation' clearly drew on long personal, cultural and historical encounters with Buddhist teachings,[14] but Kabat-Zinn's clinical programme also sig-nificantly built on modern relaxation theories and practices as popularly accepted and therapeutically understood. As he recalled:

> From the beginning of MBSR, I bent over backward to structure it and find ways to speak about it that avoided as much as possible the risk of it being seen as Buddhist, 'New Age', 'Eastern Mysticism' or just plain 'flakey'. To my mind this was a constant and serious risk that would have undermined our attempts to present it as commonsensical, evidence-based, and ordinary, and ultimately a legitimate element of mainstream medical care.[15]

In the late 1980s, the classes were reestablished in the Stress Reduction Clinic, 'emphasizing that it was a clinical service... in the Department of Medicine'. The programme was renamed 'mindfulness-based stress reduc-tion' in the early 1990s, 'to differentiate the approach from many pro-grammes that also used the term stress reduction or stress management but that had no dharma foundation whatsoever'.[16]

In today's crowded health and well-being marketplace, mindfulness has fared well by differentiating itself from other techniques that have occu-pied similar terrains. It has expanded its scientific credibility and increased its therapeutic applications, while selectively embracing its deeper Buddhist ethical framework to become embedded in a variety of clinical and non-clinical settings. Nonetheless, echoes of twentieth-century therapeutic relaxation strategies ring through recent mindfulness implementations. A recently launched mindfulness-based childbirth and parenting antenatal course, at the influential Oxford Mindfulness Centre, for example, includes 'learning how to work with pain and fear during childbirth', and 'managing stress... and other emotions, as a parent, and in everyday life'.

Recognizing the structural overlaps between relaxation and mindfulness interventions – notwithstanding their technical differences – offers impor-tant insights into why 'mind-body' therapeutic solutions to personal and social challenges are widely desired yet ambivalently received. Relaxation history elucidates the underlying socio-political conditions, and the popular and professional health and well-being ideologies, which have enabled and driven such practices to take root in our perpetually restless times.

Acknowledgements This work was supported by the Wellcome Trust [104411/Z/14/Z].

NOTES

1. 'Mindful Nation UK: Report by the Mindfulness All-Party Parliamentary Group (MAPPG)' (Mindfulness Initiative, October 2015), http://the-mindfulnessinitiative.org.uk/images/reports/Mindfulness-APPG-Report_Mindful-Nation-UK_Oct2015.pdf.
2. Compare, for example, Kabat-Zinn's widely circulated audiovisual meditation *The World of Relaxation: A Guided Mindfulness Meditation Practice for Healing in the Hospital and/or at Home* (John Kabat-Zinn, 1982), with later declarations such as: '[Mindfulness] meditation is not relaxation spelled differently. Perhaps I should say that again… Meditation is not relaxation spelled differently' (Jon Kabat-Zinn, *Coming to Our Senses: Healing Ourselves and the World through Mindfulness* [New York, N.Y.: Hyperion, 2005], 58).
3. Edmund Jacobson, *You Must Relax: A Practical Method of Reducing the Strains of Modern Living* (New York ,N.Y.: McGraw-Hill, 1934), 8.
4. See E.J. Boome and M. A. Richardson, *Relaxation in Everyday Life* (London: Methuen & Co. Ltd., 1938).
5. Ibid., 99.
6. Ornella Moscucci, 'Holistic Obstetrics: The Origins of "Natural Childbirth" in Britain', *Postgraduate Medical Journal* 79, no. 929 (2003): 168–73.
7. Original image available at Wellcome Images: https://wellcomeimages.org (search under L0079526). Image has not been modified in any way.
L0079526 Credit NCT/Wellcome Library, London, Wellcome Images Havering Branch: antenatal class photograph.
The National Childbirth Trust.
SA/NCT/B/1/2/1/3/7.
Photograph
From: National Childbirth Trust (NCT) 1952–2014
Collection: Archives & Manuscripts
Library reference no.: Archives and Manuscripts SA/NCT/B/1/2/1/3/7
Copyrighted work available under CC BY 4.0
8. See Ayesha Nathoo, 'Initiating Therapeutic Relaxation in Britain: A Twentieth-Century Strategy for Health and Wellbeing', *Palgrave Communications* 2 (2016): 16,043, doi:10.1057/palcomms.2016.43 for a deeper discussion of the gendered uptake and application of relaxation therapies; and Meyer Friedman and Ray H. Rosenman, *Type A Behavior and Your Heart* (New York, N.Y.: Alfred Knopf, 1974) for more on 'Type A' behaviour and cardiac disease.

9. Galen Ives, 'Relax', *Journal of the Royal College of General Practitioners* 28, no. 188 (1978): 187.
10. Karin Roon, *The New Way to Relax* (Kingswood: World's Work, 1951), 252.
11. Mark Singleton, 'Salvation through Relaxation: Proprioceptive Therapy and Its Relationship to Yoga', *Journal of Contemporary Religion* 20, no. 3 (2005): 289–304.
12. Geoffrey Harding, *Relaxation and Healing*, n.d., 9.
13. Herbert Benson, *The Relaxation Response* (N.Y.: Morrow, 1975).
14. On the transformation and appropriation of Buddhism and Buddhist meditation in the West, see David MacMahan, *The Making of Buddhist Modernism* (Oxford: Oxford University Press, 2008) and Jeff Wilson, *Mindful America: The Mutual Transformation of Buddhist Meditation and American Culture* (Oxford: Oxford University Press, 2014).
15. Jon Kabat-Zinn, 'Some Reflections on the Origins of MBSR, Skillful Means, and the Trouble with Maps', *Contemporary Buddhism* 12, no. 1 (2011): 282.
16. Ibid., 286–9.

Ayesha Nathoo   is a medical historian at the Centre for Medical History, University of Exeter. Her current research examines the growth of therapeutic relaxation in twentieth-century Britain, in relation to chronic-disease prevention, pain management, and health and well-being advocacy.

CHAPTER 10

So Even the Tree has its Yolk

James Wilkes

Abstract This creative-critical work draws on the archives of the Pioneer Health Centre, also known as the Peckham Experiment, held at the Wellcome Library. The Centre was established between the wars both to provide the conditions for, and to investigate, health rather than illness. The ways in which personal and group forms of vitality were conceptualized, valorized and put to work allowed poet and writer James Wilkes to think through the link between individual and societal relationships to leisure, work and health. However, the archive also holds many other strands of thinking – esoteric, biological, quasi-anarchist – and the choice of fiction as a form of writing provides a way of holding these dispersive, messy ingredients together – a way of working restlessly with restless materials.

Keywords Archival writing · Literary fiction · Peckham Experiment · Pioneer Health Centre · Wellcome Library

J. Wilkes (✉)
Durham University, Durham, United Kingdom
e-mail: wilkes_ja@yahoo.co.uk

© The Author(s) 2016
F. Callard et al. (eds.), *The Restless Compendium*,
DOI 10.1007/978-3-319-45264-7_10

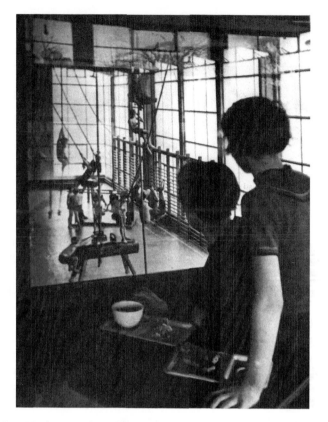

Fig. 10.1 'Mother watches while she and her daughter have their tea'. (*Source*: Wellcome Library Archive, SA/PHC/H.1/6/8. Reproduced by permission of the Pioneer Health Foundation. © Pioneer Health Foundation, released under a Creative Commons Attribution 4.0 International License (CC BY 4.0))

First visit to mother's studio in three months. She showed me the axolotls. The tank is huge, far too big for the space really, set on a trestle in the middle of the workshop. She pulled an old bed sheet off it and lit up a neon tube behind it. The light flickering through the soft grey water: like summer in Whitby. Mother has always had a theatrical streak, mostly inappropriate. I asked if the creatures wouldn't be happier in the dark but she pretended not to hear me. Three outsize newts hanging motionless a few inches above the gravel before slowly backing into the pearlescent soup. When she dropped in morsels of meat they snapped at them with sudden

twists of their necks. It's ox thyroid. I'd like to see Maggie get that from
her butcher. I pretended not to hear her. We watched the thin streamers of
blood slowly twist and disperse. You must come back in two weeks' time.

Three weeks later: mother has taken delivery of a vast quantity of
builder's sand. Bags of it are blocking the corridor and spilling over the
floor. Crunching between leather soles and plywood. I find her on a step-
ladder with a bag on her shoulder, enthusiastically tipping it into the tank.
She beckons me forward. There on a promontory of sand, clear of the
grey waters, sits a lizard. Its skin glistens darkly, and it blinks.

Eyelids! She was excited. And legs, proper weight-bearing legs. And
caudal wasting. It means the tail's become thinner. And it's not a lizard,
it's a salamander. We must be accurate.

I have a very clear image of her going for the overhaul. Rubber tubing,
and the cuff round her arm. On the workbench is the circular metal box.
I want to call it a binnacle. The Bio-Chemist looks into it. She looks
across at it and he looks down into it, directly, placidly. She has tucked
her bottom lip under her teeth, to bite and to concentrate. Brows pulled
down slightly. Showing worry or focus. And who's the girl? Leaning
against mother like she belongs here, also looking at the binnacle, wondering what's inside. The girl smiles a little. Upturn and downturn. In
the rack, five clear glass test-tubes with five clear measures of liquid,
and five dark glass bottles, unstoppered behind them. The Bio-Chemist
placid in a white coat, a pencil behind his ear. The mother lip-biting,
brows slightly drawn, a hairclip behind her ear. The girl (but where did
she come from?) interested, curious, lips curled slightly into a smile. The
binnacle we can't see into, but he can see into. He touches it lightly with
three fingers. The workbench is plain, is what she would have called deal.

I was fine until I walked into the studio. It was not knowing where to
start. The sheer quantity of stuff to be cleared and sorted. None of it inher-
itance material. My sister walked in with a box of crockery. I hope you see
that Cups and Saucers can wreck an expedition if Leaders look at cups and
saucers, I said to her. Or, and this is the new fact, engage Authoritarians to
authoritate Cups and Saucers – for sooner or later the expedition would halt
to do the Cups, and Drinking water would be used in the Desert to wash
cups! And we have several deserts to cross and few and far are the oases to
nourish us. She looked at me, her brows pulled down. We both looked side-
long at the tank under its dust sheet, relegated to the corner. I pulled the old
covering off it. Inside nothing but sand dunes stretching for miles.

The shoebox is filled with papers. One is a typescript lecture. The bottom
half of the page is composed from three separate slips, two longer and one

shorter, economically pinned together with round-headed brass pins that splay behind, the top carefully cut so it starts halfway through a line – recent developments of Medical Science – the composite whole carefully attached to its parent with one deeply rusted dressmaker's pin and one splayed brass pin. An orphan half-sentence – that divine gift, the child, is today – struck out with one line of ink. Halfway down: On the rubbish-heap of Freudianism there has fallen a seed out of which has blossomed a new valve for parenthood. On closer inspection, a single vertical line has been crossed through the second 'v' and a 'u' written in the margin. A new value. A new valve. Mother's parental instincts spurted through a hose over which she kept a firm thumb. We walked our childhoods misted in it.

Julian Huxley wrote a letter to *Nature*, January 1920: The thyroid diet began on November 30th last. On December 17th the stage which is critical in metamorphosis induced by air breathing had been passed. On December 19th the next or penultimate stage, with scarcely a trace of larval characters, was reached. The larger specimen had climbed out of the water up a platform provided for the purpose, and its skin was as dry as an ordinary salamander's.

Julian Huxley wrote a letter to the shoebox, July 1950: As regards evolution, this is only a technical term for the process of the development and transformation of life during geological time, just as ontogeny is the technical term for the development of the individual in time. Both are descriptive terms, describing processes. To say that either of them is a 'force' seems to me a most dangerous and misleading kind of vitalistic mysticism, which at all costs is to be avoided in biology.

Another sheet comes out so damp it's almost disintegrating. The fibres come away on your fingertips. Handwritten on it in a dark graphite pencil, lists of names and attributes. Jimmy Fuller: lack of muscular coordination; Harry Thomas: a certain awkwardness of gait; Herbert Fairfax: skills at woodwork; Harry Johnson: reasonably competent hairdresser; Jim Thomas: wizard with a saxophone; Herbert Winterbottom: pocket Napoleon. I see her glancing into the luminous grey waters of the tank, making notes.

We're not sure what to do about the installation of petrol cans. They make a moraine scree slope backed against one wall of the old canteen. Did she put them there or just never bother to get rid of them? When you open the door the smell: the rich turpentine that's left when volatile elements evaporate, creeping into the nostrils. She never showed us this. Maggie picked one out and looked into it. She held it up and I saw her eyes circled in red. Rusted through the base. We should throw a match into this lot. I couldn't tell if she was joking.

Seven days later: petrol cans again. In crate number four – several sheets of dry soft notepaper, covered by someone at speed, marked with paperclip rust. Because grandmother never wrote, she was the hand of choice for letters from fairies, elves, spirits. But this isn't her. Home equals something something sociological carriage of parenthood. Illegible lines. Whereas the female power, the petrol, has to be collected. Skip a bit. It has its Geometric, Earth zone, and its Dynamic or Sol zone, its Solmetricity. Parenthood the only autonomic source of geometric or dynometric something or other. Unless sustained, the battery deteriorates and the petrol-can rusts and perforates. What has happened to Society? Skip a bit. Individuals run down, their batteries are something their potential and their Petrol-cans are leaking. Why? Skip a bit. The charging station is a-virile and infertile. Illegible bit. Legible bit: We appeal not to Femininity and to Females, but to breasted women who have or feel the urge to suckle humanity, nor from the bottle, but from the breast.

In the car park we threw a lit match into one. It didn't go up like we were thinking. It seemed to go out. But then, invisible at first, a pale flame started to flicker through the holes, growing in intensity until the dented metal pinged and the valves hissed.

Two days later: the tank has been dragged into the middle of the studio and Maggie is adjusting the big halogen right over it. She's lowered the rig so the lamp is dipping into the tank. She plugs it in and a fierce glare illuminates the sand. I ask her what she's doing and she shrugs. The lamp stays on as we eat the takeaway I've brought, until the glass walls are warm to the touch. Late in the night, as we're sitting against it, warming our backs and holding up one of the photos from the shoebox, the filament goes. A loud pop and darkness and the quiet tick of cooling metal.

From up in the rafters you look down into a gymnasium-like space. Half of the back wall and all of the right is of translucent grey glass. Four – no, five – rope ladders are in motion, each with a child as a pendulum. One leans back through the ladder, toes stretched to the ground, about to kick off. One is on the bottom rung, legs tucked up, moving low and circular. One sits on the second bar, at the height of her parabola. One has his arms and shoulders through the sixth bar, toes gripping the third, the rest of the ladder flicking out beneath. One stands on the floor and holds the ladder to attention. A note on the back: Swinging not to avoid, but swinging into space.

Out of the darkness she says: salamanders communicate by opening and closing their nasal valves. She says something else about their skin that

I immediately forget. Then: this is a zone of exchange. It was in one of her letters. A place where materials are digested and exchanged. Placental. We built the workbench together. First me and her, then you and her. A workbench inside her. I can hear her uncrumpling a dry ball of paper in the night.

AFTERWORD

The Peckham Experiment, more formally known as the Pioneer Health Centre, was a social experiment into community health, and into what health and the study of health might actually mean. It was the brainchild of two doctors, Innes Hope Pearse and George Scott Williamson, and was based in Peckham, South London, between the wars, reopening in 1946 only to close for good in 1950. In its later stages, from the mid-1930s, it used a purpose-built building on St. Mary's Road, a few minutes' walk from Queens Road station, which functioned both as a community centre with a swimming pool and café, and a location for family health checks – a space in which people could use their leisure time to exercise their potential to live healthy lives.

The centre's archives are now kept at the Wellcome Library, and some very unlikely conjunctions are held together in this mass of typescript lectures, handwritten notes, early drafts of books, letters and photos. An overt commitment on the part of the founders to the 'biological' and to the study of organisms in their unconstrained environment sits alongside a covert theosophist belief in cosmic harmony; a genuine commitment to ideals of self-organization and anti-authoritarianism is paired with more discomforting elements, such as an investment in 'maternal vitality' that sometimes shades explicitly into the language of eugenics, or in esoteric images through which essential natures for men and women are imagined and brought into being through lectures, books and medical consultations.[i]

This complex, multi-faceted content demands a form of response in which diverse materials can speak to each other in multiple ways, and in which patterns, relations and contradictions can emerge.[ii] Moreover, the material qualities of the archive push certain forms of making to the fore. Most obviously collage, a process of writing that works with found material and puts its creative energies into the selection, the cut and the suture, into marking, or indeed sometimes erasing, the boundaries between registers, voices and discourses. A way of making that materially marks the

[i] See Chap. 9.
[ii] See Chap. 5.

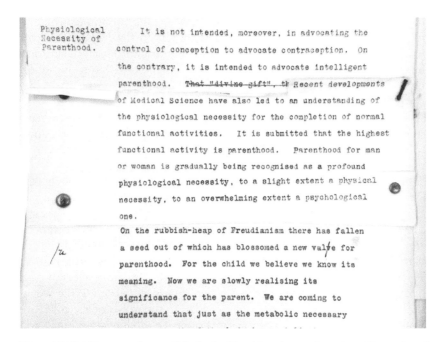

Physiological
Necessity of
Parenthood.

It is not intended, moreover, in advocating the control of conception to advocate contraception. On the contrary, it is intended to advocate intelligent parenthood. ~~That "divine gift",~~ th Recent developments of Medical Science have also led to an understanding of the physiological necessity for the completion of normal functional activities. It is submitted that the highest functional activity is parenthood. Parenthood for man or woman is gradually being recognised as a profound physiological necessity, to a slight extent a physical necessity, to an overwhelming extent a psychological one.

On the rubbish-heap of Freudianism there has fallen a seed out of which has blossomed a new value for parenthood. For the child we believe we know its meaning. Now we are slowly realising its significance for the parent. We are coming to understand that just as the metabolic necessary

Fig. 10.2 Extract from 'Medical Considerations for the Control of Contraception', p. 4. Innes Hope Pearse. (*Source*: Wellcome Library Archive, SA/PHC/E.16/1. Reproduced by permission of the Pioneer Health Foundation. Wellcome Library Archive, SA/PHC/E.16/1. Reproduced by permission of the Pioneer Health Foundation. © Pioneer Health Foundation, released under a Creative Commons Attribution 4.0 International License (CC BY 4.0))

points of indecision, change and editorial intervention, and even in some cases leaves the old versions buried under the paper, and rust spreading from the join towards the finished text.

George Scott Williamson wrote, in an incomplete letter to the General Secretary of the Family Welfare Association, that:

> [T]he ethologist or cultivator does not practice – if he exists – he is like the worms in the garden, only seen at the earliest dawn – all his work is subterranean – even his 'Casts' are anonymously swept from the 'Well Kept Lawn'. So any study of 'What's Right' is done in the dark and surreptitiously.'[1]

Literary fiction, of whatever genre, but perhaps especially the short story or prose poem which is less hostage to the expectations of plot, seems to me to be a particularly adept machine for keeping meaning turbulent, for allowing connections and narratives to perpetually reconstellate, for working in the dark and surreptitiously. I like to think that Williamson's image could be applied to writers (of any gender) as well as to his ethologists: writers as cultivators of excessive meaning, worming their way through the subsoil and ruining well-kept lawns.

But narrative is not the preserve of one discipline, and there are many stories within this archive that surface and disappear in fragmentary, unresolved ways. One such story concerns 'Little Maggie', an infant who is pinned proleptically by the title of the document in which she appears as 'The Biter'.[2] The cause for her biting is eventually located in a family psychodrama, but we never discover why she was picked out as an example, exactly what her exemplary role was, or the longer story of what happened to Maggie. We don't know what Maggie's opinions of her family's diagnosis are. This elusiveness, as well as the obvious asymmetries of power that these narratives produce, make them uncomfortable reading, and this discomfort is something else that fiction needs to work with. Beyond a self-righteous dismissal or denouncement of the way narrative is assimilated to the silencing of others, discomfortable writing can be, in the words of the collective Antena, a way to 'make us strangers in a place we thought was home', and a necessity if 'we are to imagine and begin to build a new world'.[3]

NOTES

1. 'Dear Ben', Ben Astbury, General Secretary of the Family Welfare Association (?c.1950). Wellcome Library Archive, SA/PHC/D.1/7/25.
2. Papers on family as focus of treatment. Wellcome Library Archive, SA/PHC/B.3/11.
3. Antena, *A Manifesto for Discomfortable Writing/Un Manifiesto Para La Escritura Discómoda* (Libros Antena/Antena Books, 2014), 3, 6, http://antenaantena.org/wp-content/uploads/2012/06/discomfortable.pdf.

FURTHER READING

Ginzburg, Carlo. *Threads and Traces: True False, Fictive*. Translated by John Tedeschi and Anne C. Tedeschi. Berkeley, Calif.: University of California Press, 2012.

Hall, Lesley A. The Archives of the Pioneer Health Centre, Peckham, in the Wellcome Library. *Social History of Medicine* 14, no. 3 (2001): 525–38.

Pester, Holly. *Go to Reception and Ask for Sara in Red Felt Tip*. London: Bookworks, 2015.

Pioneer Health Centre Peckham, with Papers of George Scott Williamson MD (1884–1953) and Innes Hope Pearse (1889–1978). Wellcome Library Archive, SA/PHC, n.d.

Smith, Ali. *Artful*. New York: Penguin, 2013.

James Wilkes is an Associate Director of Hubbub. He is a poet and writer, as well as a researcher at Durham University (Department of Geography). His interests range across contemporary and modernist poetry, audio and visual art, and their intersections with the life sciences.

CHAPTER 11

Cartographies of Rest: The Spectral Envelope of Vigilance

Josh Berson

Abstract For Hubbub, the anthropologist Josh Berson designed a field study with the aim of integrating physiological, phenomenological and environmental measures with place and time, and of giving study participants a chance to reflect on the experience of monitoring their movements. Here, Josh outlines how treating rest as a phenomenon with a spectral envelope emerged as a natural way to emphasize the non-linear interaction of all these factors.

Keywords City · Environmental data · Mobile sampling · Self-tracking · Spectral envelope · Vigilance

Imagine a busy urban scene – for concreteness, say Shoreditch, London, or Shibuya, Tokyo, on a Friday afternoon on the first really warm week of the year. Feel the vocal and vehicular vibrations. Every vibrating thing has a *fundamental frequency*, the lowest of the many frequency components that make up the oscillatory movement of that thing. For sounds, the fundamental frequency is that which gives us the sound's pitch, while

J. Berson (✉)
Berlin, Germany

© The Author(s) 2016   91
F. Callard et al. (eds.), *The Restless Compendium*,
DOI 10.1007/978-3-319-45264-7_11

the energy of the vibration gives us the sound's loudness. But of course there is more to sound than pitch and loudness. We have no trouble distinguishing two sounds, equal in pitch and loudness, made by two different voices or instruments. The same is true of another oscillatory phenomenon, social rhythms of activity. To describe either phenomenon we need more than the fundamental frequency. We need the *spectral envelope*.

In signals processing (the analysis of the waveform properties of a signal, that is, any phenomenon that varies in intensity in time or space, such as ambient sound pressure, respiratory volume in the lungs or the illuminance in different parts of a photograph) *spectral envelope* refers to characterizations of variation in the *mix* of frequencies present in a signal over time. Measures of a signal's spectral envelope offer a concise way to describe features of the signal that emerge from the interaction of frequency, energy and time. For acoustic signals – sounds – spectral envelope is associated with those perceptual features we subsume under *timbre*: all that is neither pitch nor loudness, things like 'brightness', 'hoarseness', 'smoothness' and 'roughness'. Timbre is that dimension of sound as a sensory phenomenon that allows us to distinguish among different voices and instruments making what, from the perspective of loudness and pitch contour, is the same sound.[i]

As Hubbub unfolded, I came to think of the task of Cartographies of Rest, the strand of the project that Dimitri Nieuwenhuizen of LUSTlab[1] and I led, as one of characterizing the *spectral envelope of vigilance*.

On the surface, our self-imposed brief could not have been simpler: *Build an instrument to measure social rhythms of rest and its opposites in the wild. Make it participatory. Make it scalable.* But responding to the brief turned out to be tricky. First, we were trying to bring together two strands of thinking with a long history of mutual distrust in anthropology: a 'constructivist' view that prioritizes the juxtaposition of incompatible ways of making sense of the world and a 'positivist' view that stresses the reduction of research hypotheses to a manageable number of measures that can be sampled efficiently in a population. Second, we were trying to bring together incompatible approaches to research: that of social science, which stresses the contextualizability, reliability and validity of measures with reference to past work (and which demands rigorous safeguards against the risk of adverse outcomes for respondents/participants) and that of human-centred design, which favours rapid iterability and user engagement over the rigour of results. Third, we were trying to operationalize a feature

[i] See Chap. 18.

of human life – restedness – that had not been adequately operationalized before, and do it in a way that would allow us to draw in a broad range of participants who would stick with us for weeks or months at a time. Finally, we were determined to break out of the paradigm that has defined mobile sampling studies up till now. This paradigm is one in which what is of interest is what is happening inside participants' bodies (as the ever-expanding number of self-tracking apps makes clear) – never what is happening in their environment or at the interface between body and world. This last challenge is where the concept of a spectral envelope comes in.

As the project went on, we came to focus more and more on sound, but my use of 'spectral envelope' here is not just about sound. Rather, what I'm trying to capture is that temporal and spatial periodicities in the collective habits of activity and mood in a population represent an outcome of how individuals interact, in dyads and groups, with one another and with a host of environmental cues, many anthropogenic, most coming under one of three broad headings: sound, light and movement. We can no more describe social rhythms of activity and rest in terms of a linear summation of individual behaviour than we can describe the timbre of a busy urban scene – recall Shoreditch and Shibuya – as a linear summation of the fundamental frequencies of the individual voices and vehicles within hearing. Instead we must look for more supple ways of capturing the many-to-many interactions among moving bodies and between moving bodies and world.[ii]

Vigilance

Why *vigilance*, as opposed, say, to *activity, alertness, wakefulness, awareness* or *arousal?* I started thinking of the phenomenon we were trying to track as vigilance in 2013, when I began turning a set of lectures I'd been giving on 'circadian selfhood' into what became the chapter on 'clocks' in my monograph *Computable Bodies.*[2] An article comparing the phenomenology and pathophysiology of mania and attention deficit hyperactivity[3] led me to a case report from the mid-1980s describing 'disturbed vigilance in mania'.[4] The report details two cases in which an individual with a history of episodic mania was admitted to hospital showing classic signs of mania – motor agitation, expansive mood and insomnia. In both cases, within minutes of eye closure, electroencephalography (EEG) showed 'sleep spindles', the characteristic brain electrical marker of the early stages of sleep. Observations of this type, difficult to reconcile with the phenomenology of mania, went largely

[ii] See Chaps. 4, 6, 7, 12.

unappreciated for decades but have lately been rediscovered. The hyperactivity and sensation-seeking characteristic of mania and attention deficit hyperactivity disorder (ADHD) represent, Hegerl and colleagues hypothesize, an effort on the part of the individual to create a stimulating environment to counteract the dangerous implications of depressed endogenous vigilance – that is, the dangers of not being aware of your environment.

Harvey, in her review of the role of circadian rhythm anomalies in mood disorders, cites the same case report and stresses the need to see circadian regulatory dysfunction as a potential cause, rather than simply a consequence, of mood dysregulation.[5] That is, disruptions in rhythms of rest and activity are not simply a symptom of an underlying mood disorder: these disruptions *may be* the underlying phenomenon. The recent dramatic rise in the incidence of recurring non-episodic mood disturbances, especially in young people,[6] may represent, in part, an outcome of dramatic changes in our social and material environment that make it difficult to establish a robust alternation of activity and rest. The timbre of our activity rhythms is getting noisier.

I came to feel that 'activity', 'arousal' and 'alertness' did not go far enough in describing what we were trying to capture in Cartographies of Rest. Our target was not simply motoricity or activity in the sense of 'activity tracker', the increasingly popular accelerometer-based devices that have become a metonym for the migration of self-tracking technologies out of the psychiatric clinic and into the realm of consumer wellness.[7] Rather, what we were after was the relationship *between* motoricity and attention. This is what I mean by vigilance.

In other words, we needed to decompose rest into at least two components. More than that, we needed to find ways of sampling these components that would allow the most diverse range of people possible – diverse in background and life history and diverse in attentional-motoric style – to provide data targeting roughly the same underlying phenomenon while at the same time allowing them to rely on their own, mutually divergent rubrics for assessing what that phenomenon entails in terms of bodily experience. 'Activity' in the sense of 'activity tracker' means something like 'whole-body motoric tonus'. This was way too coarse-grained to use as a proxy for 'activity' in the sense of 'rest–activity rhythms'.

Vigilance comes with its own conceptual baggage. The term has another, more common, sense: vigilance in the sense of preparedness or threat readiness,[8] an attunement to demands for attention and social synchronization in our perisomatic space. The two senses – preparedness and attentional-motoric tone – are related; for instance, a surplus of threat in one's environment will tend to produce a heightened attentional-motoric tone, not just in the moment but over time. Another way to put it would be to say that state vigilance – vigilance in the moment – contributes, over time, to heightened trait vigilance.

It is difficult to operationalize phenomena such as vigilance in a manner sufficiently supple for anthropological purposes, more difficult still to study them in the wild and to formulate a comparative framework, that is, to imagine a continuum of differentiated *registers* of motoricity and attention.[9] Ideally, you'd plot the spectral envelope of vigilance in a population rather than simply measure changes in individual activity level over time. This was exactly what I wanted Cartographies of Rest to do.

'NEAR SENSING' AND A PERSPECTIVAL VIEW OF URBAN SPACE

In our first pilot study, in June 2015, we sought to integrate standard physiological measures of restedness into our sampling platform. We started with heart rate variability, since reduced heart rate variability represents a widely validated measure of stress and fatigue, and a number of vendors have brought to market inexpensive, consumer-grade devices, most using a bracelet form factor, that promise to measure heart rate using ulnar photoplethysmography – optical sensing of dilation of an artery in the wrist – with strong correlation with the results you'd get using a chest strap. Heart rate bracelets proved a dead end for a bunch of reasons. For one, the wearer's movements distort the signal, and smoothing the signal to filter out motion artefacts makes the data worthless. Once the data have been smoothed, it's only valid down to a resolution of about one minute, and this is as fine-grained as device vendors will let you see. But to compute heart rate variability you need *instantaneous* resolution, that is, the time between successive heartbeats. A more serious problem was that self-tracking measures focus exclusively on events unfolding *inside* users' bodies. If you rely on these measures, you implicitly adopt a model in which the key determinants of well-being are things internal to the individual. But we wanted to incorporate social and environmental measures into our model. More than that, we wanted to make the research process itself participatory.

Participants in our first pilot – nine design students at the University of the Arts Utrecht – said that what they'd really like to have had was an opportunity to annotate their responses with audiovisual data. So in the second pilot, in November 2015 in Berlin, we included just such a feature, asking participants to include one photo and one audio sample every time

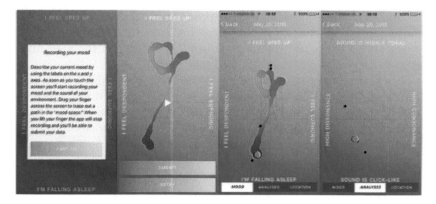

Fig. 11.1   Handset views from the Cartographies of Rest app. Once a day, users receive a notification asking them to comment on their state of being. To respond, they trace a path through a two-dimensional 'mood space'. The mood space is reliable at the individual level but provides some play for individual differences in the phenomenal coding, the 'feel', of physiological processes. While the user responds to the prompt, we record background sound. Users can review their own data and see how their data fall in the broader panel of users. Future iterations will include groups and channels that allow users to view data from just a subset of the total population of users.

we polled them. The audio samples in particular turned out to be surprisingly varied and revealing.

By pairing self-report data (see Fig. 11.1) with ambient environmental data, we could reorient mobile sampling methods away from their fixation on the autonomous body and toward a richer picture of how states of being are made through the ongoing encounter of bodies with other bodies and their shared environment. That is, we could start to treat our participant-users as social and spatio-temporal anchor points from which to look out *into* the world. I came to think of the technologies we were experimenting with not as technologies of self-tracking but of *near sensing*, by analogy with remote sensing.[10]

Once you break out of the mindset that mobile sampling is fundamentally about individual participants, higher moments in the signal that emerge from interactions among participants and between participants and their environment become more salient – that is, it becomes more natural to view the research question not in terms of the sum of individual participants' fundamental frequencies (of activity or mood or vigilance or whatever other measure) but in terms of the spectral envelope of the entire panel of participants taken as a unit.

In Haruki Murakami's *Hear the Wind Sing*, first published in 1979, the anonymous narrator pursues an experiment in self-awareness remarkably similar to those of contemporary self-trackers. He rapidly becomes disillusioned:

> I believed in all seriousness that by converting my life into numbers I might be able to get through to people. That having something to communicate could stand as proof I really existed. Of course, no one had the slightest interest in how many cigarettes I had smoked, or the number of stairs I had climbed, or the size of my penis. When I realized this, I lost my *raison d'être* and became utterly alone.[11]

The 'proof' to others that we really exist, the substance of our presence as social beings, resides not in our habits as individuals but in our collective life. To measure rest or any other dimension of well-being, we need to look beyond the skin envelope of the individual body.

Acknowledgements Thanks go to Dimi Nieuwenhuizen of LUSTlab, to Mark IJzerman for technical expertise on sound analysis, and to Felicity Callard for Hubbub leadership. The studies conducted under the aegis of 'Cartographies of Rest' received oversight from the Research Ethics Committee of the Geography Department, Durham University. For more information on the application described above, please visit http://corapp.org.

NOTES

1. LUSTlab, 'LUSTlab', accessed 26 June 2016, http://lustlab.net.
2. Josh Berson, *Computable Bodies: Instrumented Life and the Human Somatic Niche* (London: Bloomsbury, 2015).
3. Ulrich Hegerl et al., 'Are Psychostimulants a Treatment Option in Mania?', *Pharmacopsychiatry* 42, no. 5 (2009): 169–74.
4. B. Van Sweden, 'Disturbed Vigilance in Mania', *Biological Psychiatry* 21, no. 3 (1986): 311–13.
5. Allison G. Harvey, 'Sleep and Circadian Functioning: Critical Mechanisms in the Mood Disorders?', *Annual Review of Clinical Psychology* 7 (2011): 297–319.

6. Ellen Leibenluft, 'Severe Mood Dysregulation, Irritability, and the Diagnostic Boundaries of Bipolar Disorder in Youths', *American Journal of Psychiatry* 168, no. 2 (2011): 129–42.
7. Berson, *Computable Bodies*.
8. Andrew Lakoff, 'Preparing for the Next Emergency', *Public Culture* 19, no. 2 (2007): 247–71.
9. Berson, *Computable Bodies*.
10. Laura Kurgan, *Close up at a Distance Mapping, Technology, and Politics* (Brooklyn, N.Y.: Zone Books, 2013).
11. Haruki Murakami, *Wind/Pinball: Two Novels*, trans. Ted Goossen (New York, N.Y.: Vintage, 2016), 59.

Josh Berson is an anthropologist with a background in computer science and design research. He has wide-ranging interests in how culture mediates human adaptation to the world, and is the author of *Computable Bodies: Instrumented Life and the Human Somatic Niche* (Bloomsbury, 2015).

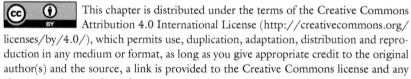

CHAPTER 12

Getting the Measure of the Restless City

Des Fitzgerald

Abstract Questions of mental health and urban life have long been central to Des Fitzgerald's research, and his work with Hubbub has led him to further explore some of the literatures and histories that undergird that relationship, and to think more expansively about the sociology of this emergent space. Critically, engagement with Hubbub has enabled contact with a range of creative practitioners (technoscientific and artistic) interested in very similar kinds of questions. This chapter outlines the development of Des's consideration of the empirics of urban ill-health.

Keywords Bodies · Environmental exposure · Interdisciplinary · Mental health · Urban

Why is it that the experience of city living is, for so many people, an experience of unease, if not illness? Why is it that a place that is for many (for *me*, most of the time) profoundly enlivening in its restlessness and its hurry, can also become, for others, an entirely overwhelming space of noise, disquiet and clamour? What is it about the urban form of life, fundamentally,

D. Fitzgerald (✉)
Cardiff University, Cardiff, Wales, United Kingdom
e-mail: FitzgeraldP@cardiff.ac.uk

© The Author(s) 2016
F. Callard et al. (eds.), *The Restless Compendium*,
DOI 10.1007/978-3-319-45264-7_12

that it associates – and has associated for some time – so strongly with the experience of mental ill health?[1]

Of course there is nothing original (to me) in such questions: as my collaborators and I have elaborated elsewhere, questions like these have concerned scholars of all stripes (as well as other writers and investigators) for more than 100 years.[2] They continue to capture scholarly and popular attention today: as I was writing this chapter, *Scientific American* published an in-depth analysis of two new studies on the association between city living and schizophrenia,[3] *Vice* carried a story on how placing trees and parks in urban neighbourhoods can have a marked effect on mental health,[4] and *The Guardian* suggested that Cardiff (my own city) was notable for having an especially high rate of panic attack.[5] Such accounts, and the studies they report on, are typical of the wider problem space of urban life and mental health; they draw on a long heritage of attempts to parse the psychogenic effects of the restless city *vis-à-vis* the calming effects of the bucolic countryside.

I take such questions of public health very seriously, and my attempts to understand this space come through a commitment to contribute to them, however marginally. That contribution is rooted in two wider concerns: (1) a theoretical attention to how bodies and societies, in some sense *get in to*, or intersect, one another – especially as such intersections take place in illness-inducing, restless spaces of noise and tumult; (2) an empirical concern with how we might come to know, to trace or to *measure* such intersections.

How, then, do bodies come to matter in urban space today? There are many ways to approach a question like this: one way, for example, would be to focus on what Josh Berson, in this volume,[i] calls 'social rhythms of rest' – and to assemble the conceptual and material tools for getting some purchase on the bodily states that emerge and disappear within specific urban rhythms. What becomes apparent, in the midst of such an endeavour, is that the question of bodies in cities is not a question of how one impacts, or has an effect on, the other: living-in-the-city is rather about being caught within a very specific set of material-semiotic relations – relations between, *inter alia*, people, bodies, brains, psyches, neighbourhoods, bureaucracies, buildings, noises and so on. To think about mental health in the restless city is to think about what happens when those relations get bent out of shape – when what comes to matter is not only

[i] See Chap. 11.

the conviviality and multiplicity of the metropolis, but also alienation and anxiety, stress and sickness. I mean 'comes to matter' here in the sense that the feminist theorist Karen Barad uses this phrase:[6] I use it in the sense of how something new (a sensation, an illness) materializes; but also in the sense of how this new thing comes to make a difference (biological, political) in the life of a citizen or of a community.

That question of making a difference also reminds us that temporality and novelty are at stake here. We have known, for some time, about the myriad ways that the social and environmental exposures of urban life bear down upon the city dweller. But we still know relatively little about how the digital and biological transformations of the *present* – which coalesce in the city, though they are not unique to it – might yet torque these exposures, as well as our responses to them. Here, again, the empirical work of Berson and his collaborators can offer some routes in: their entangling of bodily measures and self-reported ambient environmental data, for example, produces new forms of sensory intimacy with a body moving around a city.[ii] In attending to these transformations, it is also important to pay attention to other temporally complex, non-digital inhabitants (and producers) of the restless city. I think here especially of animal, arboreal and microbial life – of foxes, forests, bacteria – as these continue to make their presence felt, within the set of material relations through which urban life takes form today.[7] How this very varied patchwork of restless objects and inhabitants can be brought into some kind of synthetic understanding remains, I think, an open question.

And that question produces an ancillary problem: if we are going to learn to account for the complex ways in which bodies and cities come to inhabit one another, then it may be that what matters here is not so much theory, but measurement. How are we to bring the relationship between mobile bodies and restless cities into some kind of empirical understanding – and to do so with a view to intervening in questions of mental health, at both individual and environmental scales? A great deal of empirical work is underway: we already have, on the one hand, high-quality epidemiological attention to how the forms and stresses of urban life might produce particular symptoms and syndromes.[8] And we have, on the other hand, a potent and growing ethnographic corpus on the intersections of illness, atmosphere and place, especially as these take shape within urban and peri-urban spaces.[9] But what we lack, in the most basic sense, is a

---

[ii] See also Chap. 18.

method for working *across* these very different sets of empirical procedures. What we do not yet have is some way of accounting for the body-in-the-city that is able to attend to the two poles of that conjunction, at more or less the same time, with the same level of acuity, and the same degree of nuance, within an understanding that organisms and their environments are simultaneously (if temporarily) their own thing *and* in relation to one another at the same time.

What kinds of experiments can we imagine for opening up this space? How might we thread an ethnographic attention to place through an epidemiological concern with the specificity of diagnosis, and *vice versa*, precisely so as to mirror the cat's cradle of relations, intersections and wrappings that take place between and across cities and bodies?[10] How might we leverage precisely the same computational and digital transformations that are, as we speak, remaking a range of urban landscapes, in order to make those landscapes visible, measurable, even modifiable? These are the questions we'll need to answer, if we are truly going to get the measure of the restless city.

NOTES

1. Dana March et al., 'Psychosis and Place', *Epidemiologic Reviews* 30, no. 1 (2008): 84–100.
2. Des Fitzgerald, Nikolas Rose, and Ilina Singh, 'Living Well in the Neuropolis', *The Sociological Review* 64, no. 1 (2016): 221–37.
3. Diana Kwon, 'Does City Life Pose a Risk to Mental Health?', *Scientific American*, accessed 26 June 2016, http://www.scientificamerican.com/article/does-city-life-pose-a-risk-to-mental-health/.
4. Lucy Jones, 'Green Peace: How Nature Actually Benefits Your Mental Health', *VICE*, 24 May 2016, https://www.vice.com/en_uk/read/why-is-nature-actually-good-for-your-mental-health.
5. Amy Fleming, 'Which UK City Suffers the Most Panic Attacks?', *The Guardian*, 24 March 2016, sec. Cities, https://www.theguardian.com/cities/2016/mar/24/panic-attack-poll-swansea-most-panic-stricken-city.
6. Karen Barad, *Meeting the Universe Halfway: Quantum Physics and the Entanglement of Matter and Meaning* (Durham, N.C.: Duke University Press, 2007).
7. Robert Lee Hotz, 'Big Data and Bacteria: Mapping the New York Subway's DNA', *Wall Street Journal*, 5 February 2015, sec. US, http://www.wsj.com/articles/big-data-and-bacteria-mapping-the-new-york-subways-dna-1423159629; Jesse Ausubel, 'The Return of Nature: How Technology Liberates the Environment', *The Breakthrough*, Spring 2015,

http://thebreakthrough.org/index.php/journal/issue-5/the-return-of-naturehttp://thebreakthrough.org/index.php/journal/issue-5/the-return-of-nature.

8. Florian Lederbogen, Leila Haddad, and Andreas Meyer-Lindenberg, 'Urban Social Stress–Risk Factor for Mental Disorders. The Case of Schizophrenia', *Environmental Pollution* 183 (December 2013): 2–6.

9. Michelle Murphy, 'The "Elsewhere within Here" and Environmental Illness; Or, How to Build Yourself a Body in a Safe Space', *Configurations* 8, no. 1 (2000): 87–120.

10. Donna Haraway, *ModestWitness@Second_ Millennium. FemaleMan_Meets_ OncoMouse: Feminism and Technoscience* (New York, N.Y.: Routledge, 1997).

FURTHER READING

Adli, Madza. 'Urban Stress and Mental Health'. *LSECities*, November 2011. https://lsecities.net/media/objects/articles/urban-stress-and-mental-health/en-gb/.

Benedictus, Leo. 'Sick Cities: Why Urban Living Can Be Bad for Your Mental Health'. *The Guardian*, 25 February 2014, sec. Cities. https://www.theguardian.com/cities/2014/feb/25/city-stress-mental-health-rural-kind.

Choy, Timothy K. *Ecologies of Comparison: An Ethnography of Endangerment in Hong Kong*. Durham, N.C.: Duke University Press, 2011.

Lederbogen, Florian, P. Kirsch, L. Haddad, F. Streit, H. Tost, P. Schuch, S. Wüst, et al. 'City Living and Urban Upbringing Affect Neural Social Stress Processing in Humans'. *Nature* 474, no. 7352 (23 June 2011): 498–501.

Fitzgerald, Des, Nikolas Rose, and Ilina Singh 'Revitalizing Sociology: Urban Life and Mental Illness between History and the Present'. *British Journal of Sociology* 67, no. 1 (2016): 138–60.

Des Fitzgerald is a sociologist of science and medicine at Cardiff University, with a particular interest in the history and present of the neurosciences. He is co-author of *Rethinking Interdisciplinarity across the Social Sciences and Neurosciences* (Palgrave Macmillan, 2015).

104 D. FITZGERALD

The images or other third party material in this chapter are included in the work's Creative Commons license, unless indicated otherwise in the credit line; if such material is not included in the work's Creative Commons license and the respective action is not permitted by statutory regulation, users will need to obtain permission from the license holder to duplicate, adapt or reproduce the material.

CHAPTER 13

Drawing Attention: Ways of Knowing Derived in the Movement of the Pencil

Tamarin Norwood

Abstract This chapter explores interpretations and distortions of the visual world that occur through drawing and mind wandering. Tamarin Norwood's writing is informed by scientific literature on doodling, fidgeting, concentration and mind wandering considered in the course of her Hubbub research, and draws on chance encounters shared with collaborators in The Hub. These interactions have helped shape the imaginative approach Tamarin takes to her writing, foregrounding the possibility of movement as an impetus for generating new thought.

Keywords Blindness · Drawing · Haptic visuality · Looking · Seeing

John Berger writes: 'It is a platitude in the teaching of drawing that the heart of the matter lies in the specific process of looking. A line, an area of tone, is not really important because it records what you have seen, but because of what it will lead you on to see'.[1] Lead you on to see, or lead you on to know? Certainly the process of drawing is connected to looking, depending as it does upon a spectrum of correspondences between eye,

T. Norwood (✉)
University of Oxford, Oxford, United Kingdom
e-mail: email@tamarinnorwood.co.uk

© The Author(s) 2016
F. Callard et al. (eds.), *The Restless Compendium*,
DOI 10.1007/978-3-319-45264-7_13

object, stylus and support. But these correspondences are also home to a kind of blindness, and in my experience of drawing, the specific process of looking and not seeing is what leads you on to know. The form of knowing that emerges is restlessly attentive to the shifting terrain upon which it draws: a terrain explored not by sight but by the interplay of sightlessness, movement and touch.

I set out to draw the woodland around me and the trees come apart before my eyes. The sparse canopy overhead becomes a meshwork geometry of line, texture and gap. A horizontal array of oblongs cuts across the nearest trunks where sunlight hits. It draws a line across the scene, connecting the elbow of a distant trunk, a prominent crop of foliage in the foreground, a thickening of branches towards the right edge of the copse and what might be a figure at work in the distance, near the low horizon. The illuminated trunks become margins that edge patches of deep irregular shade, which in turn present their own geometries: this one almost triangular, this one almost rectangular, this one almost the inverse of that one and so on. The more I look to draw, the less I am able to see the thing I had once seen – a glimpse of springtime woodland in the late afternoon sun – as it becomes subtly different: an observed version of itself, an object, an objectified thing.[i]

Such is my experience every time drawing begins. The looking and plotting that happens just before I set pencil to paper, and which continues as drawing goes on, is a kind of restless seeing allied to not seeing and to blindness. I want to examine the dynamics of this restlessness by comparing three distinct images from art history, film theory and anthropology, which together locate the practice of drawing at the intersection of perception and locomotion.

Drawing has been associated with not seeing since its mythical origin in the ancient Greek story of Butades, the potter's daughter who sets out to draw her lover to capture his likeness before he leaves, turning away from him to trace his shadow on to the wall. But her action precipitates his departure, her physical turning away embodying a conceptual turning away that takes place through the act of drawing. By regarding him from a vantage point from which she can capture his likeness, she initiates his withdrawal into objecthood: a withdrawal that draws forth a trace or shadow left behind as a signal of his absence. What she finally draws is not him but his shadow, not the reality of the man but the idea of him,

[i] Cf. Chap. 4.

projected on to the clay like the shapes that dance inside Plato's cave. It is 'as if seeing were forbidden in order to draw', as Jacques Derrida writes in his treatise on blind drawing, 'as if one drew only on the condition of not seeing'.[2]

So, the act of drawing begins by throwing everything into the dark, and the stylus moves forward into this darkness, on to the page, its movement breaking a path where before there was nothing. Derrida imagines what the stylus might see, pressed so close to the page, and finds it deeply myopic. From the 'aperspective of the graphic act', the stylus is blind both to the form that precedes it (the thing it sets out to draw) and the form that follows it (the drawing that will appear on the page), and instead sees nothing but the immediate present of its 'originary, path-breaking moment'.[3] As he constructs an analogy between drawing and blindness, it is striking that he writes less about the absence of sight than the presence of movement and touch. It is not simply that drawing is blind, but that the stylus is a 'staff of the blind' that 'feels its way', providing a tactile proxy for sight; and that the fingertips grope about the page 'as if a lidless eye had opened at the tip of the fingers, as if one eye too many had grown right next to the nail, a single eye, the eye of a Cyclops or one-eyed man'; this lidless eye being, moreover, 'a miner's lamp' whose light makes inscription possible.[4] Throughout his account of blindness, the conflation of movement, touch and sight is never out of reach. As I draw the woodland, my eyes move fractiously about the fragmented scene before me while my pencil moves likewise about the page, so that touch becomes a close proxy for sight. Movement and touch turn out to be integral to the forms of seeing, not seeing, knowing and not knowing that drawing brings forth. This dynamic is exposed in a second image, this one from film theory, which presents seeing without seeing, or seeing by touch, as a strategy for coming to know.

Haptic visuality is a way of looking in which the eyes behave like fingertips, brushing or caressing the surface of the thing seen;[ii] a mode of visuality that has much in common with Derrida's complex of blindness, near-darkness, closeness, and his conflation of sight and touch. Film theorist Laura Marks explores examples of film and video that court this way of being watched. In *Seeing is Believing* (1991), a video by Shauna Beharry,[5] a photograph of a piece of fabric is filmed at very close quarters. The closeness means the shot is often out of focus, and is very dark when the lens makes contact with the photograph. When the image is dark, it becomes grainy and doubly hard to see. Watching the video, explains Marks, one is primarily aware of surfaces: of the lens, the photograph and the fabric, and of the screen upon which the video plays (indeed, Marks's book is titled *The Skin of the Film*). Reflecting upon her own experience of watching the video, she writes: 'I realize … I have been brushing the (image of the) fabric with the skin of my eyes, rather than looking at it'.[6] In Marks's account, the aperspective of the haptic look is coaxed forth in films and videos that obscure or obstruct vision in one way or another, often through graininess, darkness and lack of focus. These interventions make the viewer vividly aware that whatever is being watched is being watched and caught on film, and moreover that the act of watching and capturing on film is precisely what obscures the thing from sight. The near conflation of these surfaces, each pressed so close to the next, means there is never enough distance to see the whole of any object or indeed to make out surface detail, to understand its topology, or to apprehend the trail the camera lays along its surface. Unlike Butades' gaze, which for Derrida seeks to capture the thing it sees and succeeds in pushing it away, the haptic look brings with it a way of knowing that, by moving with and along the thing it regards, inspires 'an acute awareness that the thing seen evades vision'.[7] This closeness of touch recalls the probing of the stylus as it makes its way along the surface of the page drawing its object into being, and it suggests a way of coming to know that depends not only upon contact but upon movement. What form of knowing is made possible by the movement of the stylus in drawing?

A third image, that of a wayfarer laying a trail along the surface of a terrain, elaborates this possibility. Anthropologist Tim Ingold provides an account of the dynamics of wayfaring that has much in common with the movement of the haptic lens, and with the 'cautious and bold' creeping forward of the blind men who people Derrida's essay and who 'must advance' bodily through space in order to discover what lies ahead.[8] For the wayfarer, as for the stylus, lens or figure who gropes in the dark, movement proceeds by means of continuous contact with the terrain, the intimacy of this contact supplying the perceptual clues necessary for advances to be made:

> Proceeding on our way things fall into and out of sight, as new vistas open up and others are closed off. … Thus the knowledge we have of our surroundings is forged in the very course of our moving along them.[9]

What Ingold would call the bond between locomotion and perception yields in drawing 'a form of knowledge that is activated or emerges simultaneous to the situation …, a way of knowing the world that cannot be transferred or banked, nor accumulated into the knowledge of the encyclopedia'.[10] This description, by the artist Emma Cocker, derives from drawing experiments which emphasize in particular the restlessness of the drawing act. Cocker elicits from the act of drawing a form of knowledge that is vigilant to the changing conditions of the terrain it explores, 'feeling its way [and seizing] opportunities made momentarily visible'.[11] The form of knowing that emerges in time with the movement of the pencil is forged in the course of this movement and – like a wayfarer foraging for nourishment in the environment around – it is even sustained by it. Drawing depends upon constant, moment-by-moment attentiveness to the changing contingencies of the drawn form as it arrives on the surface of the page; each change in tone, density, direction, velocity feeding the next.[iii] From the aperspective of the graphic act, to know what lies ahead one must physically move ahead, laying a trail that creates and is created by the richness, complexity and unpredictability of the surface. This is a kind of tactical knowledge 'capable of responding to situations which are contingent, shifting or unpredictable', pushing forward into the unknown and 'producing what is unknown' by these means.[12]

Through these three images (the stylus, the camera lens and the wayfarer), remaining restlessly attentive and vigilant to the blindness inherent in drawing emerges as a strategy for knowing *with* the thing being drawn, rather than seeking to know it or know about it. Here I intend the word 'with' both in the sense of a mutual engagement, and in the sense of employing the thing being drawn as a strategic means for advancing into new knowledge – working with it as one works with a tool. As the pencil moves about the page attentive to the object it draws into being, what appears is not a drawing of the woodland but a drawing with the woodland: a drawing that employs the woodland to create something entirely new that could not have been created without it. The specific process of looking and not seeing is one of close, tactile engagement quite unlike Butades' experience of turning away and tracing a shadow. A proxy for my unseeing eye, the pencil moves about the paper as though it moved about the surfaces of the trees themselves, laying down marks like caresses that acknowledge their touch as the

---

[iii] See. Chap. 11.

very thing that makes the woodland inaccessible to sight. Finally, what I come to know about the woodland by drawing it is that I do not know it. The marks left on the surface of the page are an expression of, and consolation for, the loss of the thing I have drawn away by setting out to capture it on paper.

NOTES

1. John Berger, 'Life Drawing', in *Berger on Drawing*, ed. Jim Savage (London: Occasional Press, 2007), 3.
2. Jacques Derrida, *Mémoires d'aveugle: l'autoportrait et autres ruines* (Paris: Éditions de la Réunion des Musées Nationaux, 1990), 49.
3. Ibid., 45.
4. Ibid., 51, 4, 4.
5. Shauna Beharry et al., *Seeing Is Believing* (Montréal, Québec: Groupe Intervention Vidéo, 1991).
6. Laura U. Marks, *The Skin of the Film: Intercultural Cinema, Embodiment, and the Senses* (Durham, N.C.: Duke University Press, 2000), 127.
7. Ibid., 191.
8. Derrida, *Mémoires daveugle: l'autoportrait et autres ruines*, 5.
9. Tim Ingold, *Lines: A Brief History* (London and New York: Routledge, 2007), 87–88.
10. Emma Cocker, 'The Restless Line, Drawing', in *Hyperdrawing: Beyond the Lines of Contemporary Art*, ed. Phil Sawdon and Russell Marshall (London: I. B. Tauris, 2011), xiv.
11. Ibid.
12. Ibid., xvii.

FURTHER READING

Detienne, Marcel, and Vernant, Jean-Pierre. *Cunning Intelligence in Greek Culture and Society.* Chicago, Ill.: University of Chicago Press, 1991.

Hull, John M. *Touching the Rock: An Experience of Blindness.* 1990. New edition, London: SPCK, 2013.

Nancy, Jean-Luc. *Le plaisir au dessin.* Paris: Editions Galilée, 2009. [*The Pleasure in Drawing,* translated by Philip Armstrong. New York, N.Y.: Fordham University Press, 2013].

Schwenger, Peter. 'Words and the Murder of the Thing'. *Critical Inquiry* 28, no. 1 (2001): 99–113.

Tamarin Norwood is an artist and writer working with text, video and sculptural installation. She has recently completed commissions for Tate Britain, Art on the Underground and Modern Art Oxford, and through 2016 is artist-writer in residence at Spike Island (Bristol).

CHAPTER 14

Songs of Rest: An Intervention in the Complex Genre of the Lullaby

Holly Pester

Abstract This essay is the product of thinking, researching and singing lullabies. As a practitioner-researcher in Hubbub, Holly Pester led a series of workshops that experimentally and collaboratively explored lullabies through conversation and improvised song. This led to an expanded project where Holly invited artists and musicians to collaborate on a collection of new lullabies, created through friendship and improvisation. The thoughts and provocations within this chapter represent the politics and ideas that have motivated this project.

Keywords Care · Creative criticism · Lullaby · Narrative · Protest song · Reproductive work

1.

Who is the traditional singer of lullabies? We instinctively want to say mothers and to consider the lullaby in terms of the intimate bond between mother and child. But the practice of lulling the baby to sleep in a family or community unit falls along distinct lines of labour relations and cultures of social reproduction. Lullaby singers are those who nurse, heal, craft and care, those who 'invisibly' produce the

H. Pester (✉)
University of Essex, Colchester, United Kingdom.
e-mail: hpester@essex.ac.uk

© The Author(s) 2016
F. Callard et al. (eds.), *The Restless Compendium*,
DOI 10.1007/978-3-319-45264-7_14

economy,[i] infrastructure and ecology of the home. Who is the traditional singer of lullabies? The mother, the sister, the maidservant, the nanny, the wet nurse and colonized bodies of imperial systems; commoning women, those whose work is turned into capitalized care and that in turn supports work outside the home and global economies. This is the starting point from which I have been thinking about lullabies: before their form, sound and style, I've considered the contingent politics of the lullaby and how the principles of care, from a socio-historical standpoint, and from within the cult of the family, are carried through in their singing.

My mother could not give me a boy as good as you

2.
The sound of lullaby is the cry of reproductive work. The lullaby is the mother's (the sister's, the maidservant's, the nanny's) work song. Like any shanty or marching chant the rhythms of her body and the tempo of the song – rocking and jigging the baby into slumber – co-ordinate the act of material effort (in the scene of supposedly immaterial labour). Here, as with washing, cooking, loving, sympathizing, comforting and breast-feeding, the woman's body performs as a resource to soothe and oil the mechanics of capital.[ii] This is care work shown for what it is, sweating, muscular movement-task.

How long have we been not at work, in rest space?

3.
What narratives are sung in a lullaby? The scenarios range across universes, realities and times: baby-stealing fairies, cursed soldiers, murder ballads, angered house demons, father-killing hyenas, sunken ships. But the imperatives to sleep are expressed through certain identifiable categories. They can be defined as: shush, there is work to do and tasks that need to be completed, things that need to happen and can't until you are asleep; if you don't sleep I will curse you, this is my threat, this lullaby is my spell; hush now, imagine this radically different space and hear this surreal story that bears no familiarity to our lives. It is not a question of the baby understanding these narratives or even comprehending the need

[i] See Chap. 20.
[ii] See Chap. 16.

for it to sleep, but it is the singer's (cultural) compulsion to voice their anxieties, frustrations, fears and dreams. The song ritualistically blesses/ curses the social relations and economic conditions of the family.

I can't begin to tell you, how tired I am

4.
The comfort of the lullaby is not just its cradling rocking back and forth with the hushing tones of the voice. It is the comforting of the 'social factory' where everyone is where they should be (*Father's gone a-hunting*), the divisions of labour are being met (*Mother's gone a-milking*), and the order of production (*Sister's gone a-silking*) and the cogs of capital (*Brother's gone to buy a skin*) are melodically soothed.

Small life rooms, small life rooms, small life rooms

5.
While these systems of labour coalesce in the song, what gets produced by the work of the song itself is a slumbering baby. In other words, what gets produced by this work song is a state of inactivity. The lullaby, therefore, is a complex of labour relations and affection as well as a dynamic of work and non-work, effort and rest. The lullaby is dependent on the work of one body for the rest of another. Within the dynamic of the cradle song, one resisting body transforms into stillness, muscles calm, bones relaxed. The other body, resisting tiredness, works at calming the active and vigorous form. It is a focused task, tiring and difficult, and one of the last of the day. From this dialectic of effort and slumber at play in the lullaby, we might say that it produces an 'other' to work rather than its opposite.[iii] The other to work being a form of active resistance to work logic that in itself requires effort, while the opposite is a ceasing of work and effort. From this reclaimed perspective we might also see the potential in lullabies to problematize the principle of work as productivity.

Tonight you might feel your feet multiply

6.
So if there is something that provokes non-work in the lullaby, can it be harnessed as a protest song? Can a lullaby sing in resistance to work and

[iii] Cf. Chap. 17.

can it be a song of people subjected to the technologies and ideologies of capitalism? (The 8-hour day, the 7-day week, the market's appropriation of bodies for the production of its workforce.) And are there commonalities and solidarities that the lullaby can sing to other forms of night labour – beyond the excesses of the working day, to the bodies that toil outside that frame – and to other forms of care?

Rainbows and horses, these are my causes, little bear

7.

If we relocate the lullaby, seeding it outside the mainstream family scene, what are the possibilities for it to become a song of radical care? First we should ask: Through the act of lullabying, what other agencies, critical of existing forms of social reproduction, can play out? Can we use the lullaby to sing out an economy of care that is (genuinely) outside, or other to, the systems that resource labour and reproduce social conditions?

When you come home signing, I'll come home singing

8.

While the lullaby is a conduit to slumber, we might find a form or practice of lullaby that is not for soporific effect, but which gifts permission to stop, to become other-to-work. The lullaby might affectively perform a common rest. If a lullaby sounds out the material labour of care, makes its flesh and breath felt, then it can also sound out the halting, obscuring, decentering, dismantling of work, as an active resistance.[iv]

split, shift, split, shift, split, shift, work

9.

Who cares?

Children and young carers, those caring for the elderly (unsettling and reversing the affect flow of the lullaby).
Friends (the alternative to family, the alternative economy).
Animals (humans for animals, animals for humans, animals for animals).
Those engaged in the restitution of mental illness, care workers, aid givers, and sanctuary and shelter workers.

[iv] See Chap. 21.

Lovers (the sexual, affective, emotional labour of being a lover).
Political allies (solidarity and community, struggle).
Migrant domestic workers (those whose care work is dependent on their disenfranchisement).
What do the lullabies of these relationships sound like? What narratives are coded into them?

Low low low low low low low ... go on

10.
The ultimate anticapitalist, antifamily lullaby is Woody Guthrie's 'Hobo's Lullaby'.[1] We find out that it isn't actually the song that's the lullaby, but the sound of the boxcar where the hobo sleeps. It is the mechanical sound of the margins, beyond the home, work conditions and fixed labour roles. This is a lullaby of movement – the struggle for comfort, the comfort of the struggle. The condition of the hobo's body, soothed by the train carriage, itself a cog of moving capital, is as much produced by socio-economic conditions as it is extrinsic to them. This paradoxical slumber is an other to work. The work of being a hobo ('I know the police cause you trouble, they cause trouble everywhere') is other to systematized labour. This lullaby acknowledges the violence and pain of this condition as it sings its radical potential.

NOTE

1. Written by Goebel Reeves.

FURTHER READING

Federici, Silvia. *Revolution at Point Zero: Housework, Reproduction, and Feminist Struggle*. Oakland, Calif.: PM Press, and Brooklyn, N.Y: Common Notions and Autonomedia, 2012.

García Lorca, Federico. 'On Lullabies'. In *Deep Song and Other Prose*, edited and translated by Christopher Maurer, 7–22. New York, N.Y.: New Directions Publishing Corporation, 1980.

Leslau, Wolf. 'Inor Lullabies'. *Africa: Journal of the International African Institute* 66, no. 2 (1996): 280–87.

Holly Pester is a poet working in experimental forms, sound and performance, and an academic at the University of Essex (in Poetry and Performance). Her work has featured at Segue (New York), dOCUMENTA 13 (Kassel), Whitechapel Gallery and the Serpentine Galleries (London).

CHAPTER 15

Could Insomnia Be Relieved with a YouTube Video? The Relaxation and Calm of ASMR

Giulia Poerio

Abstract Giulia Poerio's public engagement work with Hubbub has featured her psychological research on autonomous sensory meridian response (ASMR) – relaxing, tingling sensations that start at the top of the head and spread down the neck, spine and sometimes throughout the rest of the body, usually in response to certain triggers. Giulia's collaborative studies aim to examine the self-reported and physiological correlates of ASMR experience.

Keywords Autonomous sensory meridian response · Relaxation · Self-report data · Synaesthesia · Well-being

Recent figures suggest that over half of Britons have trouble getting to sleep at night.[1] If, you, like so many other people, struggle to nod off,

G. Poerio (✉)
University of York, York, United Kingdom
e-mail: giulia.poerio@york.ac.uk

© The Author(s) 2016
F. Callard et al. (eds.), *The Restless Compendium*,
DOI 10.1007/978-3-319-45264-7_15

119

then you may have tried various strategies to slip into a peaceful slumber – from classic remedies such as warm milk, a hot bath or a consistent bedtime routine to the more unconventional, such as cherry juice, acupressure, or sleep shots containing an ostensibly sleep-inducing cocktail. But what if watching a particular kind of YouTube video could relieve insomnia? Millions of people are avid viewers of ASMR YouTube videos, which promote feelings of calm, relaxation and well-being. ASMR stands for autonomous sensory meridian response and describes a relaxing, tingling sensation that starts at the top of the head and spreads down the neck, spine and sometimes throughout the rest of the body. Although many people report experiencing ASMR in response to certain triggers (e.g. whispering and tapping) since childhood, the past decade has seen a growing number of YouTube videos dedicated to inducing ASMR in viewers for rest and relaxation. For many, these videos can provide a much-needed antidote to insomnia, stress and even relief from depression and anxiety.[2] ASMR videos are eclectic, but examples include: towel-folding tutorials, simulations of haircuts, massages and medical examinations, careful dissections of fruit and vegetables, the squishing of packets of Haribo sweets, and the fondling of bubble wrap. In this chapter, I describe what ASMR is and track the emergence of both the sensation and the online community over the past decade. I argue that we now need scientific research into the phenomenon and suggest how this could be achieved by drawing parallels with research on synaesthesia.

THE UNEXPLAINED FEELING: WHAT IS ASMR?

ASMR occurs in response to certain triggers that involuntarily elicit a tingly, relaxing and pleasant feeling. Although people's specific ASMR triggers are idiosyncratic, there appear to be a number of common ASMR audiovisual triggers, which include: whispering, soft speaking, tapping, scratching, crinkling, slow deliberate hand movements, watching repetitive tasks being completed and close personal attention. In a Hubbub public engagement event at Wellcome Collection in London, we invited members of the public to watch one of ten ASMR YouTube video clips and report on their experience of ASMR. A summary of the results from the 91 people who took part is displayed in Fig. 15.1. Over half the people asked reported experiencing ASMR. Although this may suggest that ASMR is prevalent, the high rates of ASMR in this sample may be biased (e.g. people who experience ASMR may have been more likely to take part).

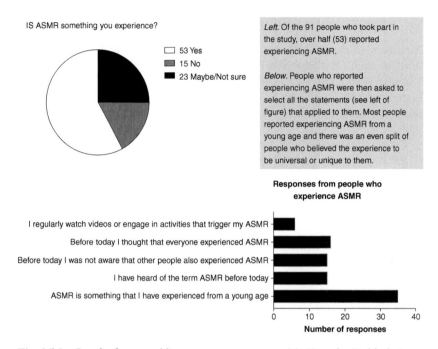

IS ASMR something you experience?

☐ 53 Yes
▨ 15 No
■ 23 Maybe/Not sure

Left. Of the 91 people who took part in the study, over half (53) reported experiencing ASMR.

Below. People who reported experiencing ASMR were then asked to select all the statements (see left of figure) that applied to them. Most people reported experiencing ASMR from a young age and there was an even split of people who believed the experience to be universal or unique to them.

Responses from people who experience ASMR

I regularly watch videos or engage in activities that trigger my ASMR

Before today I thought that everyone experienced ASMR

Before today I was not aware that other people also experienced ASMR

I have heard of the term ASMR before today

ASMR is something that I have experienced from a young age

0   10   20   30   40
Number of responses

Fig. 15.1 Results from a public engagement event on ASMR at the Hubbub 'Late' at Wellcome Collection, September 2014

Discussions with people at events such as these indicate three broad reactions to ASMR. Some people know exactly what the ASMR feeling is (although they are not always familiar with the term 'ASMR'), can recount various experiences of ASMR, and often report experiencing it from childhood. People in this category typically express one of two reactions to finding out about ASMR: surprise that not everyone has the experience (believing it to be universal) or relief to know that they are not the *only* person to experience the feeling. Sometimes people who have tried explaining the feeling to others report negative reactions, leading them to believe that they are somehow 'abnormal'. Other people categorically do not experience ASMR, often find it bizarre and can find watching ASMR videos uncomfortable (e.g. see reactions to ASMR videos).[3] A third reaction is uncertainty as to whether one does experience ASMR; ASMR, here, is typically likened to similar (but not identical) sensations, such as the chills that accompany certain songs and moments of inspiration.

THE RISE OF ASMR

Members of the ASMR community have linked certain literary descriptions to their own experiences of ASMR, quoting from, amongst others, Virginia Woolf and Sylvia Plath. I found a more recent description reminiscent of ASMR in Stephen Kelman's *Pigeon English*, which describes the sense of relaxation from watching a task being completed carefully:

> I couldn't concentrate because I wanted to see what Poppy was doing. She was painting her fingernails. She actually used the paint for pictures to paint her fingernails with. I watch her the whole time. I couldn't even help it. She painted one fingernail green, and then the next one pink again, in a pattern. It took a very long time. She was very careful, she didn't make a single mistake. It was very relaxing. It made me feel sleepy just watching it.[4]

Both literary descriptions such as these and anecdotal reports suggest that the experience currently described using the term ASMR is not 'new'. It is, however, relatively new to the mainstream media and online community. The growing awareness of ASMR within popular culture has been largely due to YouTube, the online ASMR community (on various online forums such as Reddit), and 'ASMRtists' who create video content for people to induce ASMR. The first online descriptions of ASMR appeared on various forums (e.g. SteadyHealth.com and IsItNormal.com) from 2007 where people explained and discussed their ASMR experiences. In 2009, the first ASMR YouTube video was posted by WhisperingLife who, based on her own experience of relaxation through whispering, decided to create whisper videos for others to enjoy. The rise of YouTube videos was accompanied by a subreddit in 2011 called 'ASMR. Sounds that feel good'.[5] Journalists soon noticed the growing online ASMR community and the first of many news articles on ASMR was published in 2012.[6]

Figure 15.2 shows the upsurge of interest in the term 'ASMR' using Google Trends.[7] Since 2011, interest in the topic has risen dramatically. As an example of the popularity of ASMR, the most prolific ASMRtist on YouTube (GentleWhispering) had, in June 2016, over 650,000 subscribers and her most popular video had over 15 million views. As these figures show, the interest in and widespread use of ASMR is not trivial. Simple whispering videos have evolved into realistic role-plays,[i] which

[i] See Chap. 16.

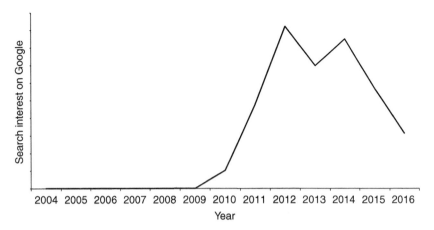

Fig. 15.2 Interest in the term 'ASMR' over time, using Google Trends (which analyses the amount of Google searches over a period of time); search done May 2016

simulate ASMR-inducing scenarios such as getting a haircut, attending medical examinations and receiving makeovers, massages or suit fittings. ASMR videos have become increasingly professional, with many ASMRtists recording with binaural microphones and high-tech audiovisual equipment. Some ASMRtists have created a 360 degree ASMR experience using 3D virtual reality; others conduct one-to-one Skype sessions for personalized ASMR; there is even an ASMR treatment spa. More recently, ASMR has been a source of inspiration for Pepsi and Dove/Galaxy advertisements, and has been incorporated into modern electronic music. I would argue that ASMR is more than just a bizarre internet craze that will subside over time: its appeal and continued growth is likely to reflect the fact that ASMR is a physiologically rooted experience, and one that people will be continually motivated to pursue.

THE SCIENCE OF ASMR

Despite widespread media attention, ASMR has gone virtually unnoticed by the scientific community. In March 2015, Barratt and Davis published the first exploratory survey (using an online questionnaire) of 475 people who experience ASMR.[8] Their results indicated that the majority of respondents had first experienced ASMR when they were between five and ten years old; 98 per cent found ASMR videos relaxing; 82 per cent and 70 per cent used the videos for sleep and stress relief respectively; and 80 per cent reported a positive effect of ASMR on mood. The most common ASMR triggers were whispering, personal attention, crisps sounds and slow movements. These results provided the first documented evidence consistent with anecdotal reports, and made the first step towards legitimizing ASMR as a scientific topic.

Despite this initial research, the ASMR phenomenon awaits more rigorous enquiry. In particular, research is needed that examines both ASMR experiencers and non-experiencers to quantify different reactions (physiological, neural, self-reported) to ASMR content. For the phenomenon to be scientifically validated, gathering more 'objective' evidence for ASMR, rather than relying purely on self-report data, is crucial.[ii] Research would profit from examining the physiological responses (such as heart rate) that accompany the ASMR experience, as well as its neural basis. Such research would provide much needed evidence for the proposal that ASMR is a phenomenon associated with a distinct and reliable pattern of physiology. However, acceptance of ASMR into mainstream psychological science is likely to be difficult, because the experience is not universal, does not have an established research base, and there may be scepticism around what the feeling is and whether it is amenable to scientific investigation. In the next section I argue that ASMR, much like anything else, is open to scientific investigation. One way to motivate and conduct research in the area is to link the ASMR experience to other accepted and similar phenomena and the research methods to investigate them; here I discuss synaesthesia as a pertinent example.

TASTING WORDS: IS ASMR A SYNAESTHETIC EXPERIENCE?

Synaesthesia, like ASMR, is a sensory experience that only some people have. It describes a 'crossing' of the senses where a sensation in one modality (e.g. seeing the letter 'A' – called the inducer) is automatically accompanied by, or elicits, an experience in another modality (e.g. seeing the colour red – called the concurrent). The most common forms of synaesthesia involve associating days and graphemes with colour. Other forms of synaesthesia include: sounds with touch, words with tastes, tastes with shapes and pain with colours.[9] Paralleling ASMR experiencers, synaesthetes

---

[ii] Cf. Chap. 6.

express surprise upon learning that others do not share their merging of the senses, such is the primacy of their own perceptual experiences.

Synaesthesia has important parallels with ASMR. To the extent that ASMR involves audiovisual stimuli eliciting a tactile sensation and feeling of relaxation, it can be conceptualized as a synthetic experience – specifically, as a form of touch and/or emotion synaesthesia. Sound – touch synaesthetes report different sounds triggering tingling/prickling sensations in different body parts; mirror – touch synaesthetes report feelings of touch/pain/emotions that mirror another person's experience (e.g. seeing somebody being hit on the head elicits the same sensation in the perceiver); and touch – emotion synaesthetes report certain textures evoking different emotions. Similarly, ASMR triggers (inducers) typically elicit tactile, tingling sensations on the top of the head, as well as associated feelings of calm and relaxation (concurrents). The link between inducers and concurrents in both ASMR and synaesthesia also appears to occur automatically and involuntarily. However, a point of difference between ASMR and synaesthesia is that, in ASMR, a wide range of triggers (e.g. whispering, tapping and close personal attention) elicit the same feeling across many different people, whereas in synaesthesia, different triggers elicit different responses and these responses differ between synaesthetes (e.g. the word 'family' may taste like a ham sandwich, whereas the word 'six' may taste like vomit). One possibility is that ASMR is a more common but as yet undocumented synaesthetic experience in which there is greater consistency among experiencers with respect to inducers and concurrents.

Aside from the notable parallels between these experiences, the development of the scientific study of synaesthesia and its acceptance into mainstream psychological science may suggest that the science of ASMR is not only possible, but also likely. Unlike the relatively new surge of interest in ASMR, synaesthesia has been documented for over 200 years, with the first scientific reports dating back to 1812. Advances in methods to document the existence of synaesthesia (such as neuroimaging and extensive testing of synaesthetic experiences)[iii] have meant that, particularly over the last 30 years, synaesthesia has been recognized as a subjective experience with a distinct physiological and neural basis, one which can facilitate our understanding of normative perception and neural development.[10]

[iii] Cf. Chap. 2.

PEOPLE FIND IT HARD TO BELIEVE THINGS THAT THEY DO NOT EXPERIENCE

ASMR is only beginning to emerge into public awareness, but there is hope that its scientific journey will follow the same historical path as synaesthesia. The first step in this journey is likely to be the dispelling of scientific scepticism around the existence of ASMR. ASMR is not something that everyone experiences, meaning that some people find it hard to believe. Scepticism is a common problem with non-universal or unusual experiences. This issue may arise because people typically generalize from their own experiences; something that is not part of our experiential world is harder to accept as true. There are many examples of this 'false consensus' effect or 'typical mind fallacy'. Would you believe that some people can recall every moment from their lives in the minutest detail, that some people do not experience any form of visual imagery, or that some people are visited by terrifying 'shadow men' intruders at night while paralysed and unable to act? These are all examples of scientifically documented experiences (hyperthymesia,[11] aphantasia[12] and sleep paralysis[13]) that, although atypical, are considered legitimate experiences for scientific study.

ASMR is fascinating whether you experience it or not. It is clear from the sheer volume of YouTube videos and associated viewing figures that it is by no means a niche experience. Anecdotal reports suggest that ASMR may offer potential to serve as a sleep aid, and a method of promoting well-being. What is essential, however, is the need to test anecdotal reports with systematic scientific enquiry, something that I and my research team are continuing to do. The onus will be on researchers to establish the physiological and neural underpinnings of ASMR, since this would demonstrate that ASMR is a reliable phenomenon in those that experience it. Once ASMR has been established as a scientific object of enquiry, it would then be possible to examine it in more detail – including exploring its origins (proximal and distal causes), concomitants and consequences, as well as its potential therapeutic and clinical benefits for rest and relaxation.

NOTES

1. Sleepio.com, 'The Great British Sleep Survey', n.d., http://sleepio.com/2012report/.
2. Rhys Baker, 'I'm Using My Newly Discovered ASMR To Fight Depression', *Thought Catalog*, 9 March 2015, http://thoughtcatalog.

com/rhys-baker/2015/03/im-using-my-newly-discovered-asmr-to-fight-depression/.

3. For example, Kirsty Liddle, 'ASMR News: YouTubers React To ASMR', *Asmryouready*, 21 April 2016, http://www.asmryouready.com/asmr-news-youtubers-react-asmr.

4. Stephen Kelman, *Pigeon English* (Boston, Mass.: Houghton Mifflin Harcourt, 2011), 45.

5. 'ASMR. Sounds That Feel Good – Reddit', accessed 20 May 2016, https://www.reddit.com/r/asmr/.

6. Nicholas Tufnell, 'ASMR: Orgasms for Your Brain', *Huffington Post*, 26 February 2012, http://www.huffingtonpost.co.uk/nicholas-tufnell/asmr-orgasms-for-your-brain_b_1297552.html.

7. Datasource: Google Trends, accessed 20 May 2016, www.google.com/trends.

8. Emma L. Barratt and Nick J. Davis, 'Autonomous Sensory Meridian Response (ASMR): A Flow-Like Mental State', *PeerJ* 3 (2015): e851.

9. For a review on synaesthesia, see Jamie Ward, 'Synesthesia', *Annual Review of Psychology* 64, no. 1 (2013): 49–75.

10. Ibid.

11. Brandon A. Ally, Erin P. Hussey, and Manus J. Donahue, 'A Case of Hyperthymesia: Rethinking the Role of the Amygdala in Autobiographical Memory', *Neurocase* 19, no. 2 (2013): 166–81.

12. Adam Zeman, Michaela Dewar, and Sergio Della Sala, 'Lives without Imagery – Congenital Aphantasia', *Cortex; a Journal Devoted to the Study of the Nervous System and Behavior* 73 (December 2015): 378–80.

13. J. A. Cheyne, S. D. Rueffer, and I. R. Newby-Clark, 'Hypnagogic and Hypnopompic Hallucinations during Sleep Paralysis: Neurological and Cultural Construction of the Night-Mare', *Consciousness and Cognition* 8, no. 3 (1999): 319–37.

FURTHER RESOURCES

The videos of GentleWhispering, the most popular ASMRtist can be found at: www.youtube.com/user/GentleWhispering (additionally, a simple search of the term 'ASMR' in YouTube will provide thousands of videos).

A website dedicated to reviewing and sharing ASMR-related resources: www.asmrr.org.

General ASMR news: http://asmruniversity.com/blog.

BBC Radio 4 documentary ('Brain Tingles') on ASMR: www.bbc.co.uk/programmes/b06s9rzk.

Giulia Poerio is a psychologist at the University of York. She researches the socio-emotional functions of daydreaming and mind wandering, and the under-studied phenomenon of autonomous sensory meridian response (ASMR, also known as 'Brain Tingles').

CHAPTER 16

Relief from a Certain Kind of Personhood in ASMR Role-Play Videos

Emma Bennett

Abstract The writer Emma Bennett first heard 'ASMR' (autonomous sensory meridian response) mentioned during interdisciplinary conversations about lullabies and the politics of work and rest while at Hubbub. After Googling the practice, Emma began watching Olivia's Kissper ASMR to aid sleep and to indulge a long-held susceptibility to 'tingles'. Here, Emma asks: Could this spectatorial practice aimed at attaining a dreamy, sleepy passivity be reframed as an active research practice? And, might this counterintuitive move raise productive theoretical questions about activity and passivity, questions that open on to the ethics of rest and its opposites?

Keywords Address · Apostrophe · Autonomous sensory meridian response · Body · Performance · YouTube

1.
Our encounters take place in a vague but easily imagined context. A room, domestic yet anonymous. A feeling of the door being closed. Not secretive so much as legitimately, respectfully private. Perhaps there isn't even

E. Bennett (✉)
Queen Mary University of London, London, United Kingdom
e-mail: e.l.bennett@qmul.ac.uk

© The Author(s) 2016
F. Callard et al. (eds.), *The Restless Compendium*,
DOI 10.1007/978-3-319-45264-7_16

a door? There wouldn't need to be one, not now I am here. In any case, I can't turn my head to look. My perception of this space is ever so slightly blurred at the edges.

Welcome, she says, *you are just on time.*

Smiling. Her face fills my vision. She looks into my eyes, and she looks at my eyes. She speaks to the space where my face would be.[i]

I can help you with your migraines, she says, *but first we will have to do some examination that will include checking your face and your facial muscles.*

As she says this she brings both her hands to her own face – she touches it twice, indicatively, symmetrically, with perfectly straight fingers.

So let me get started, she says. *I'll just gently touch your face.* Her hand comes towards me. Fingertips blur as they appear in my vision close up.

I'll just gently bring pressure on your cheeks, she says, *and the area of your jaw.*

Her gaze is fixed somewhere below my eyes, as her thumbs and fingers move at the outer edges of … what? My vision? Or my face? The four corners of it – upper eyebrow, lower jaw – drawn or dabbed gently on to the space between and in front of us. It's a mime, this momentary touch, but she definitely has nice fingers.

This is Olivia: her face, her hands, in detail, close up.[ii] The shadow on the inside of her right eye is violet, underneath it a little smudge of purple. I am looking at this stylish eye smudge, which is deliberate, like all her movements, and she's making something about the space between and in front of us palpable, shapely. Of course, she's an image on a screen: an inscription. And she's stroking not my face, but my computer screen from the inside. But I strongly feel the contiguity of our rooms, hers opening on to mine with this as the window – *this*, my screen, my face.

2.

Olivia has called this video 'CLOSE UP Medical DOCTOR Role Play'.[1] This is a mutual performance. A two-sided role play. I can see her but she can't see me. She pretends to see me: This is how it works. She looks intently in my direction, and I feel that gaze, tangibly, on my face. She

[i] Cf. Chap. 19.
[ii] Cf. Chap. 15.

is smiling, but serious, and speaks with the calm, attentive expertise of a medical professional. But the glasses she is wearing are too big; they keep slipping down her nose. A reminder that her seriousness, although it is earnest, is not entirely serious.

It is not only her performance, it is mine, too. I have to go along with it, even just a tiny bit, for it to work. I have to receive these recorded, mediated attentions *as if* they were really directed at me, personally, in the here and now. And it works: when Olivia says, *I'll just gently touch the area of your jaw*, my jaw responds, it feels noticed. It's sort of like it blushes, flinches ticklishly at the mention of its name.

With the serious, scientific-sounding term 'autonomous sensory meridian response' (ASMR) in mind, I read that, in biology, an autonomous response 'usually refers to an involuntary motor reflex such as breathing or vomiting directed by the spinal cord that is not processed by the brain'.[2] Is this an accurate way to describe what is happening when Olivia says *your jaw*, and my jaw tingles in response? In other words, is my jaw's response 'autonomous'? Is this something my jaw does *on its own*? It somehow feels that way, but cannot be, for it is the *verbal* cue that calls my jaw into play. Olivia's spoken words are what allow me to imagine and thus feel *as if* certain parts of my face are being, or about to be, touched. And, as one who thinks with and through performance, my interest lies precisely in the 'as if . . .' and the creative and theoretical space it opens. For me, ASMR is less a question of biological autonomy than linguistic agency – of a body felt, a self experienced, through language.[iii]

She pretends to see me, speak to me. I pretend she is examining me, that when she says *you*, she means *me*. And yes, when she says *your jaw*, I feel as if my jaw is playing along too, imagining itself to be another jaw, the one Olivia is imagining, fictionally examining. The whole thing relies on a deliberate confusion between the somatic and the linguistic, the willed and the involuntary, self and body, person and thing.

3.

Pitched somewhere between a careful ritual and a routine check-up, the 'close personal attention' explicitly offered by ASMR videos is reassuring precisely inasmuch as it is *im*personal. Olivia dedicates her gestures not to a named person (this would be distractingly specific), but, repeatedly, to

---

[iii] Cf. Chap. 7.

'you'. It is her repeated refrain, *this ... for you*. When she introduces into the frame a stack of cotton wool pads in a half-deflated polythene tube, uncrumpling gently, pulling out its tiny frayed drawstring, for the sound, she will say *I have this cotton wool for you*.[3]

The philosopher Adriana Cavarero calls attention to the second-person pronoun, and in so doing, subtly critiques conventional ways of understanding sociality. The 'you,' she writes, 'is a term that is not at home in modern and contemporary developments of ethics and politics.'[4] Individualist doctrines celebrate the 'I', collective movements the 'we'. Devoid of the fullness of self-assertion or the positive connotations of friendship, community and political solidarity, 'you' can tend to get overlooked. An empty, contentless indicator, it marks the destination of any address whatsoever. A 'you' might be imaginary or deferred. It could be anyone or no one. It designates a gap to be filled, nothing more.

Cavarero proposes a relational ethics that starts with the question: 'Who are you?' As Judith Butler notes, 'This question assumes that there is an other before us whom we do not know and cannot fully apprehend.'[5] Olivia's 'you' is not 'me', never quite; it just coincides with the space that I am, for this time. This is not a scary or unhappy interpellation, because not only is it explicitly provisional, it's also full of reassurance. *You have a beautiful scalp, very symmetrical, very smooth*, says Olivia, as she speaks into being a person-shaped space, a body devoid of the distracting specifics of 'me'.

4.

In her video called '1 Hour FACIAL Spa BLISS', Olivia proffers an array of little vessels and products and curiously textured items, selected *for you*, and for their sound. Each thing is held up between thumb and forefinger, carefully introduced, displayed, tested out, tapped and sounded out. Salt crystals, for example, tipped gently into a small bowl.

And I will be mixing this for you here, she says, *in this cute little container, and I will be using this stick*, tap-tap of nail on stick, *for the mixing, and this one is made of bamboo*.

For little articulations, attentions like this, they rely on sensitive microphones, which pick up surface-level meetings between the body and the things it touches. Finger pads, for example, ever so slightly moist, adhering momentarily to the tacky plastic of a travel-sized shampoo bottle, to make a gentle *thuck–thuck*. This miniaturization of attention is both pedantic and luxurious: a feeling of glazed pleasure, a passive sort of enchantment.

Videos like this are recorded using 'binaural' equipment: two micro-phones shaped like human ears, and spaced accordingly, in order to capture sound in three dimensions. When I listen, with in-ear noise-can-celling speakers, it's as if I insert my head into that space, the space Olivia describes with her words and gestures. Where the video camera is con-cerned, there is not quite such a snug fit between my own sensing appa-ratus and the recording equipment. At the scene of recording, there is an eye-like lens; at the scene of spectating, a screen. This is the window *through* which I look, and *on to* which Olivia projects my entire face.

Amongst the unresolved issues of the ASMR role-play video, particu-larly of the face-touching variety: Where is my nose? Does it float transpar-ently in the middle of my face/screen? Or should it be located somewhere unseen, off the lower edge, below my line of sight? Different ASMR artists have devised their own ways around this predicament. Olivia will say *and now I'm just going to do your nose*, and at the same time stroke, say, a cotton wool pad (freshly moistened in splashy, ceremonious fashion, with fragrant rose water) in a vertical line down the middle of the screen. *Ah*, some part of me thinks, *that's surely not where my nose is, would be, should be; surely that's the middle of my ... eye?*

Tricky moments such as this do not, for me, ruin the effect of the role play. I find the mediated encounter intensely lovely not in spite of these wonky conceits, but *because* of them. The representational conventions of the ASMR role-play are not quite established, still buzzing around the edges, and I like those moments when the joins are visible because they intensify the intimacy, the sense of colluding in a fiction.

5.

When I am watching Olivia, I am participating in the fiction, the role-play. (Although it doesn't look much like 'participation', what I am doing here, horizontal and limp-limbed, staring into a screen.) Of course, I am aware, as she knows I am, that she is, in fact, speaking not to 'me' (or anybody's body or face) but to a camera and a microphone. Her performance of care, tending the body and its parts, is directed towards this hardware, these devices.

In poetry or rhetoric, the direct address of an absent, or indeed an inan-imate, being is named 'apostrophe'. As when Yeats, for example, intones 'O chestnut tree', or Shelley 'O wild West Wind'. The term 'apostrophe' is, according to Barbara Johnson, 'based etymologically on the notion of turning aside, of digressing from straight speech', and 'manipulates the I/ thou structure of direct address in an indirect, fictionalised way'. She calls it 'a form of ventriloquism' whereby the speaker throws not only their voice, but also human form into the addressee, 'turning its silence into mute responsiveness'.[6]

Olivia's spoken performance is directed – intently, exaggeratedly – towards me, the mutely responsive viewer. But, in her room, my proxy is a technological assemblage, a camera plus binaural microphone. And so there is something simultaneously voyeuristic and thingified about this position. I am looking out from the position of the *thing* Olivia once addressed *as though* it were a person, a human being with a face. Here a curious doubling takes place: a thing is being addressed as if it were a person, and via the mediation of a screen, a digital interface, a person (me) can experience this address from the position of the thing. This might explain what I feel to be an odd displacement of my personhood, I am being addressed *as if* I were a person, but my position, my viewpoint, is that of a thing.

6.

Why is this so nice, the feeling of this uncertain status *between* personhood and objecthood? Could it be that it offers a relief from a certain kind of personhood? Projecting oneself outwards into space, into social space, can be exhausting, perhaps increasingly so in the performance-driven economy of late capitalism, where the kind of work to which we are encouraged to aspire is not that which produces material goods, but that which delivers services and creates and maintains social networks.[7] [iv] Against this backdrop, it might well be that the embodied social acts of projecting one's 'self' out towards others – smiling, speaking, comporting one's body in relation to others, turning one's face to the world – feel increasingly *like work.*

Is this what, for me, makes the address of the ASMR role play restful, relieving, *over and above* those real-life caring encounters it imitates?[v] At the doctor, the spa, I may be granted a degree of anonymity (these professional carers do not *know* me), but I am still taxed with the effort of *acting like a person,* projecting some coherent image of myself. But here, with Olivia, who promises me, amongst other things, *a peel-off mask,* a loose personhood is projected on to me by someone who cannot even see my face. This intervenes in the projecting of a coherent, bounded, personness outwards into the world; here is someone projecting a neutral and impersonal personhood (as in, human shape, human form) *on to* me.

[iv] Cf. Chaps. 8, 14, 20 and 22.
[v] Cf. Chap. 9.

When Olivia says, *you have a beautiful scalp, very symmetrical, very smooth,* and somewhere off-screen, her fingers find my hairline with a dry grassy sound which reminds me my skull is there, and also not there, I am her 'you', spoken into place. I hover between states. My body is imaginary (to Olivia) and irreducibly here (in my room, on my bed). I'm doubled, folded over and pleasantly displaced. This is how it feels, I think, to feel (and luxuriate in) what it is to be *a* 'you'. No 'you' in particular, *this* given you, the one that happens to be the object – the much-prized object – of this occasion of address.

NOTES

1. Olivia's Kissper ASMR, 'CLOSE UP Medical DOCTOR Role Play: Binaural ASMR EXAMINATION with CRANIOSACRAL THERAPY for Migraines', 11 February 2015, https://www.youtube.com/watch?v=Nyz0TRPWEag.
2. Quoted in Joceline Andersen, 'Now You've Got the Shiveries: Affect, Intimacy, and the ASMR Whisper Community', *Television & New Media* 16, no. 8 (2015), 687; see also Chap. 15 of this volume.
3. Olivia's Kissper ASMR, '1 Hour FACIAL Spa BLISS: Binaural ASMR Role Play with Sugar Scrub & Relaxation Music', 12 June 2015, https://www.youtube.com/watch?v=Viy8TRtAWQw.
4. Adriana Cavarero, *Relating Narratives: Storytelling and Selfhood* (London and New York: Routledge, 2000), 90.
5. Judith Butler, *Giving an Account of Oneself* (New York, N.Y.: Fordham University Press, 2005), 31.
6. Barbara Johnson, 'Apostrophe, Animation, and Abortion', in *The Barbara Johnson Reader: The Surprise of Otherness*, ed. Melissa Feuerstein, Bill Johnson González, Lili Porten and Keja Valens (Durham, N.C.: Duke University Press, 2014), 218.
7. For more on this, see Michael Hardt, 'Affective Labor', *Boundary 2* 26, no. 2 (1999): 89–100.

Emma Bennett performs, writes and makes recordings – working with language, voice, sound and objects. She is interested in figures of speech, obstacles and involuntary acts. She has recently performed at Santozeum Museum (Santorini, Greece), FIAC (Paris) and Wellcome Collection (London).

PART III

Practices

CHAPTER 17

R-E-S-T and Composition: Silence, Breath and aah…[Gap] Musical Rest

Antonia Barnett-McIntosh

Abstract Antonia Barnett-McIntosh's compositional concerns lie in the specificity of sound gestures and their variation, translation and adaptation, often employing chance-based and procedural operations. In this chapter, Antonia describes how her research with Hubbub investigated musical rest and its opposites, silence and noise, and rest and exhaustion, and outlines the compositional processes at work in the development of two pieces composed during her residency: *Breath* for solo alto flute (world premiere by Ilze Ikse at the Hubbub Late Spectacular at Wellcome Collection, 4 September 2015), and *none sitting resting* for string quartet (world premiere by Aurora Orchestra at BBC Radio 3's 'Why Music?' at Wellcome Collection, 26 September 2015).

Keywords Compositional practice · Flute · Performance · Rest · String quartet

A. Barnett-McIntosh (✉)
Berlin, Germany
e-mail: a.barnettmcintosh@gmail.com

139

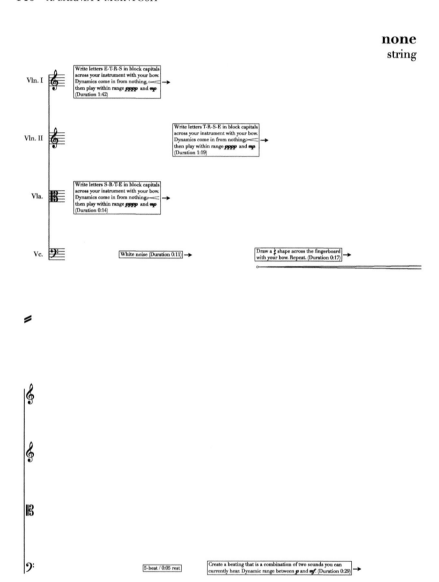

Fig. 17.1 Opening page of *none sitting resting* (*Credit:* Antonia Barnett-McIntosh, 2016)

sitting resting
quartet

Antonia Barnett-McIntosh

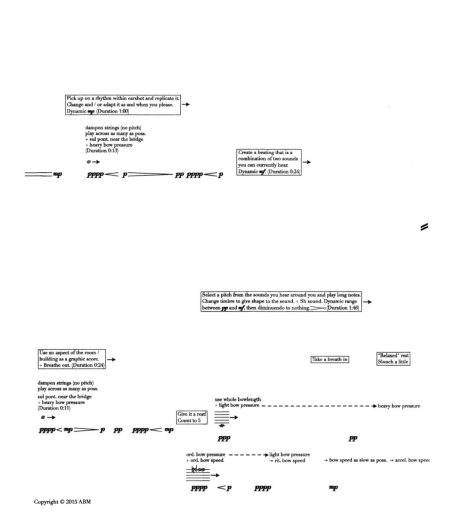

Fig. 17.1 Continued

Intro

During my research with Hubbub, I contemplated relating music to the themes of rest and its opposites. What does musical rest entail? What could the opposite of rest in music mean? What are the qualities of sound at rest in music and music notation? How could one perform rest? Simply, the first two queries suggest silence and sound,[1] and so I pondered silence....

The closest I've come to a silent experience, lengthy silence, took place above a remote New Zealand mountain-top's tree-line on a still day.[i] Above the trees, above the birds. In a musical setting, a more momentary silence occurs when a hush descends on an audience before an orchestra begins a piece (the conductor poised with baton in the air to ready the orchestra) and remains after (the conductor poised again with baton in the air, which is then released to signal the orchestra to relax).

I view silence and sound not as a binary positive/negative, but as presence and absence. Where sound exists, so does silence: They permeate each other. Musical rest corresponds to sound: preceding, proceeding, creating space in the middle, as a counterpart, creating context. Thomas Clifton writes: 'To focus on the phenomenon of musical silence is analogous to deliberately studying the spaces between trees in a forest: somewhat perverse at first, until one realizes that these spaces contribute to the perceived character of the forest itself, and enable us to speak coherently of "dense" growth or "sparse" vegetation. In other words, silence is not nothing. It is not the null set.'[2] I centred my research on looking at (listening to) those in-between spaces, between the trees, so to speak, and thinking of rest conceptually. I abstracted aspects of musical rest and recontextualized them as sound objects.

Compositional Process (and Themes of Rest)

When I begin a new piece, I imagine a page's whiteness as silence, the blankness as space mapped in time. I carefully choose gestures to position within that time-space, thinking of silence as the frame in which to place sound in a context.

---

[i] Cf. Chap. 18.

I start with pencil and paper, but even if you set the minutes of your score in notation software, bars and bars of rest appear for pages and pages laid out before you:

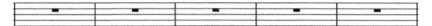

I use meditation-like tactics[ii] to confront the empty time-space, letting ideas bubble leisurely in the back of my brain. I recently began using my own version of Julia Cameron's 'Morning Pages'[3] technique (stream-of-consciousness writing by hand, first thing in the morning, three sides of A4) to help me formulate artistic concepts. Analogue writing generates ideas I wouldn't otherwise conceive by only thinking.

These words behave as prompts, triggering thoughts for what I want, and also weeding out what I don't want a piece to deal with. I can capture certain ideas and make decisions without the pressure of thinking in finished thought. I can tether multiple concepts to focus on exactly which combinations interest me. Through committing words to paper, I eliminate superfluous elements and concentrate on important ones. This writing style enables me to articulate and realize ideas casually and encourages a concept to *pop*.

The pages often establish a list of parameters first. The string quartet pages started: 'A string quartet. Around 15 minutes long. Performed in September by players from Aurora Orchestra....' You get the idea. I labelled those pages 'String Quartet brain vomit'.

A few steps later, I plan a system to generate material using a method I call my bag process. I break down into categories aspects of sounds I want to investigate. I write variables within these categories on small pieces of paper, fold them, put them into categorized bags and then 'pull' the composition by drawing out the pieces of paper. All the categories combine to create particular notes, sounds or gestures. I call on past iterations of this process to see what has worked before and tailor the current composition accordingly. This process is at once chance based and a well-considered procedure, a kind of Choose Your Own Adventure.[iii] Occasionally, I circumvent the process, depending on which combinations are possible, or not.

[ii] Cf. Chap. 9.
[iii] Cf. Chap. 19.

Categories can include instrumentation, pitch, rhythm, techniques, articulation, dynamics, duration and more. Instrumentation is usually decided for me. For a category like dynamics, I'll select a range and write out each variable within that range. Techniques and articulation depend on instrumentation, and I calculate choices based on the quality of sounds I'd like to use. Others, like pitch, rhythm and duration, can take on a random system, in which I trust my brain to come up with what I need, writing the variables on to the pieces of paper off the top of my head, as a gut reaction. I sit with a pile of pieces of cut-up paper and I get in the zone and just go for it, until I've composed the allotted time-space. As I go, I record everything I've pulled, in order, in a chart.

BREATH: A SOLO ALTO FLUTE PIECE

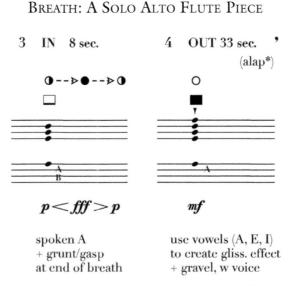

Fig. 17.2   In-Breath 3 and Out-Breath 4 from *Breath*. *Credit*: Antonia Barnett-McIntosh, 2016

In first-year composition class, our teacher played a flute piece and afterwards asked what we could say about the performer. I was struck by how little we'd noticed. I'd carefully listened to what I thought of as the composed music, not the performance. On second playing, I heard the subtle intakes of breath and realized the performer was a woman. Since then I've been interested in the in-between sounds that contribute to a performance.

For a flute player, the breath holds the pace of musical life. Reading a rest in flute music traditionally signifies the end of a phrase, at which point the performer uses the opportunity to take a breath. Breath control becomes extremely important, and flute players train for years to make breath sounds inaudible, especially when they need to take a breath quickly. Flute players have formidable stamina and lung capacity, naturally employing tactics to cope with exhaustion.

I was interested in what happened when the traditional in-breath/ out-breath structure broke, and in how I could repurpose the in-between breath as a performative sound element – as the backbone of the piece and sole source of sound, rather than a by-product. I decided to write a piece exploring the breath and rest, breathlessness and exhaustion, in which the performer utilizes each in- and out-breath in the creation of sound, exposing the inhale as an equal partner to the exhale. I asked the flute player Ilze Ikse to collaborate on the piece, and together we investigated how she could handle not taking a breath for ten minutes. We measured the lengths of her breath and experimented with adding sonic techniques. In order to literally embody the sound, the alto flute behaves as a resonator for Ilze's body and breath.

The score defines each inhale and exhale as a single gesture (Figs. 17.2 and 17.3). I constructed these using my bag process. For each one, I notated duration, airflow (open or restricted throat and variables in between), embouchure (open or closed mouthpiece and variables in between), fingering (not to denote pitch but to optimize the resonance of the sound – whether a particular construct required a more open or more closed resonator), dynamic and technique (such as using the voice, singing, speaking, sss-ing, fff-ing, whistling).

The character of the breath transforms with each gesture and the performer must concentrate on combining all the variables, which often contend for priority. In a way, I'm deliberately wishing for, prescribing, failure. The performer shouldn't appear to present an unrehearsed or badly performed piece, but the quality of the sound I'm proposing lies in the attempt to achieve these combinations, and in this case, the qualities inherent in a particular kind of exertion.

The performance of *Breath* comprises other uncertainties. One performer's capabilities and breath supply differ from another's. The playing of the piece can also depend on how much the performer slept the night before, what they ate for lunch and how nervous or relaxed they feel, for example. I'm very open to these shifting variables becoming a part of the piece. Each *Breath* performance will be a unique rendition, personal to the performer.

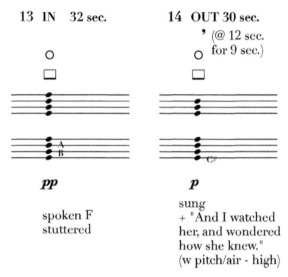

Fig. 17.3   In-Breath 13 and Out-Breath 14 from *Breath. Image* (*Credit:* Antonia Barnett-McIntosh, 2016)

NONE SITTING RESTING: A PIECE FOR STRING QUARTET

While composing *none sitting resting* (see Fig. 17.1), I worked alongside collaborators from the neurosciences, the social sciences, psychology and other artistic disciplines. And while the piece doesn't illustrate scientific ideas, my collaborators' concepts and processes permeated my work and feature in the music. For example, I borrowed the title from a poem by James Wilkes, which he generated using a linguistic corpus, a database of written and spoken language samples. James had searched the term 'resting' and the corpus returned a spectrum of English sentences containing 'resting'. I chose the shortest, 'none sitting resting'.

none sitting resting investigates the qualities of sound at rest in music and music notation. The piece comprises different concepts of musical rest. I divided the material into three main categories – musical gestures, text instructions and bow techniques. I used my bag process to generate gestures one by one. I allocated durations to each, and placed them one after another, either horizontally (in time) or vertically (in combination with other instruments). After attributing other techniques and dynamics to sculpt each gesture, I added in some 'restful' gestures – using musical rest, performed rest, pauses, gaps, breaks ('take a sip of water'), audible breath, bodily rest ('slouch a little'), one bow length as one breath, the scrapes and scratches that happen inadvertently between sounds – as sonic material for the piece.

This score is task- or action-based, rather than results-based. Again, in-between sounds play a role – the attempt to combine particular bow techniques with impossibly soft dynamics, for example – and so the overall quality of sound becomes not polished and perfected but emerges from the playing style, which adds a certain liveness in performance. One task requires that the players write capital letters from the word R-E-S-T across their instruments' fingerboards. Another asks the players to respond to sounds and visual shapes in the surrounding space (by adding a texture, selecting a pitch, replicating a rhythm) from each other's playing, or from inside and outside the performance space ('use an aspect of the room/ building as a graphic score').

The piece's length ranges between 12 and 18 minutes. I have not supplied metronome markings or accumulative time frames. Players can interpret the time-space layout of the score (where one system, or half page, could constitute roughly one to one-and-a-half minutes) as a guide. While timings have been allocated to some gestures, stopwatches must not be used. Players should estimate durations in the moment while performing, and interact with each other (though never through physical, gestural conductor-type cues), giving a sense of time stretching and contracting. This allows for numerous potential interpretations – of the sound quality of the musical gestures, text instructions and bow techniques, and of the durations of the 'restful' gestures. The performance directions state: 'Take your time. It doesn't matter if it seems like you're out of time. There's no such thing.'

Outro

Notes

1. Much writing and analysis exists on the musical function of rest and silence. If you're interested in reading more on the topic, see John Cage, *Silence: Lectures and Writings* (Middletown, Conn.: Wesleyan University Press, 1961); Zofia Lissa, 'Aesthetic Functions of Silence and Rests in Music', *Journal of Aesthetics and Art Criticism* 22, no. 4 (1964): 443–54; Jennifer Judkins, 'The Aesthetics of Silence in Live Musical Performance', *Journal of Aesthetic Education* 31, no. 3 (1997): 39–53; David Metzer, 'Modern Silence', *Journal of Musicology* 23, no. 3 (1 July 2006): 331–74; and Elizabeth Hellmuth Margulis, 'Silences in Music Are Musical Not Silent: An Exploratory Study of Context Effects on the Experience of Musical Pauses', *Music Perception: An Interdisciplinary Journal* 24, no. 5 (2007): 485–506; and Elizabeth Hellmuth Margulis, 'Moved by Nothing: Listening to Musical Silence', *Journal of Music Theory* 51, no. 2 (2007): 245–76.
2. Thomas Clifton, 'The Poetics of Musical Silence', *Musical Quarterly* 62, no. 2 (1976), 163.
3. Julia Cameron, *The Artist's Way: A Spiritual Path to Higher Creativity* (Los Angeles, Calif.: Jeremy P. Tarcher/Perigee, 1992), 9–24.

Antonia Barnett-McIntosh is a composer and sound artist. Her work has been performed in the United Kingdom, Europe, Scandinavia, New Zealand and the United States – including at Wigmore Hall and The Pit, Barbican Centre (London), Arnolfini (Bristol) and DAAD Galerie and Theater im Aufbau Haus (Berlin).

CHAPTER 18

Metrics of Unrest: Building Social and Technical Networks for Heathrow Noise

Christian Nold

Abstract This chapter describes Christian Nold's research with Hubbub, which started with working around Heathrow Airport in London and encountering the way local people are affected by the noise there. To understand the controversies concerning the impact of aircraft noise at Heathrow, it is necessary to understand the way technical metrics can systematically exclude the experience of local people. Christian seeks to address this exclusionary combination of technology and politics by building a new noise-monitoring network for Heathrow that engages equally with the social and technical aspects of noise and sees them as fundamentally intertwined.

Keywords Airport · Interdisciplinary · London · Participatory · Prototype · Sound

The problem of aircraft noise at Heathrow Airport in London dates back to the introduction of turbojet aircraft in 1958. Today, noise is still the key issue at the centre of discussions about possible airport expansion through a third runway. While proponents argue that expansion is needed

C. Nold (✉)
University College London, London, United Kingdom
e-mail: christian@softhook.com

© The Author(s) 2016
F. Callard et al. (eds.), *The Restless Compendium*,
DOI 10.1007/978-3-319-45264-7_18

149

to support growth,[1] opponents argue that it will dramatically increase air and noise pollution for local residents.[2] For politicians, the decision on whether to expand is seen as a 'toxic dilemma'[3] that is likely to alienate large parts of the electorate. As the impact of noise on human health extends well beyond hearing loss, to include increased risks of hypertension and heart disease, in addition to sleep disturbances (including daytime sleepiness), this is also a significant public health issue.[4,i]

Despite this political dilemma, the governance of noise at the airport has not really changed for the last 50 years. It is focused on a 'community annoyance' metric that quantifies the impact of noise on local residents. The current metric was created in 1982 and is based on interviews with just 2,097 residents who were asked how bothered they were by noise in the area, on a scale from 'very much' or 'moderately' to 'a little' or 'not at all'. This stated level was compared to measured sound pressure to create a curve relationship between people's stated experience and sound pressure. Based on this relationship, a threshold was identified at 57 dB LAeq, 16h, which was said to represent the 'onset of significant community annoyance'.[5] This threshold was then plotted as a contour around the airport. People living within the contour band are said to be affected by aircraft noise, for purposes such as subsidized sound insulation, while those outside it are not. Crucially, the number of people living within the annoyance contour is a key battleground in the debate over whether Heathrow should be expanded. If it can be demonstrated that the number of annoyed people would not change or might go down with a third runway, then support from the politicians is more likely to be forthcoming.

Yet many residents are extremely frustrated with the way this metric flattens and marginalizes their experience.[ii] A particular point of contention is the way the metric *averages* noise peaks, and does not represent the disruptiveness of very loud aircraft every 90 seconds. The 2M group of local authorities also argues that the current annoyance metric systematically excludes nearly a million residents who are actually affected by aircraft noise.[6] 'Member of the Public 16' provided the following stakeholder response to the Airports Commission discussion paper:

> Heathrow are also exploiting the 57 dB noise threshold to make it look like there is a reduction in noise with an expanded airport. The reality of course

[i] Cf. Chap. 12.
[ii] See Chaps. 6 and 11.

is that noise continues to be hugely disturbing to many people considerably below that threshold, me included. Where I currently live whilst better than Kew (hence I moved here) and just outside the 57 dB contour is still disturbing enough to wake my children regularly.[7]

Even acousticians agree that these annoyance metrics are out of date, largely arbitrary and merely a convenient way for governments to deal with the political problem of noise. Many residents have expressed a desire for a grass-roots process to document the reality of the noise. While there is a well-organized and active Heathrow noise pressure group called Heathrow Association for the Control of Aircraft Noise (HACAN), its focus has been on opposing expansion using political and economic arguments rather than focusing on noise monitoring. The problem is that the official hardware used for static noise monitoring is extremely expensive, and out of the reach of a distributed community noise-monitoring network. This has meant that some residents have privately paid companies to carry out a noise survey of their home. Unfortunately, these surveys have usually been short term and not had any political impact. What is missing is an independent noise-monitoring network focused on Heathrow Airport.

For the last two years I have been organizing just such a sound-monitoring network to engage with the challenge posed by the current noise metrics. The immediate goal has been an experimental network of prototypes that could function as an exemplar and encourage others to build a large-scale network with many devices and participants. The long-term goal is to set up a public process of developing an alternative metric that could take better care of the experience of local residents.

Building the network involved creating institutional relationships with Windsor and Maidenhead Council and the pressure group HACAN, both of which gave strategic advice and put me in touch with their members. It also involved public workshops and events to engage Heathrow residents in brainstorming and co-designing concepts, hardware and software. In the workshops, participants experimented with prototype devices and discussed new approaches for dealing with the annoyance metric. From these workshops the main conclusion was the need to build a network that would represent the diversity and multiplicity of noise impacts. Based on these observations, I extended the network to include sound artists and academics working on the effects of noise on biodiversity.

The hardware prototype that emerged from this process is a small computer with a calibrated measurement microphone (Fig. 18.1). People who feel they are affected by aircraft noise can place the device in their garden to measure and broadcast the impact of noise (Fig. 18.2). The device is

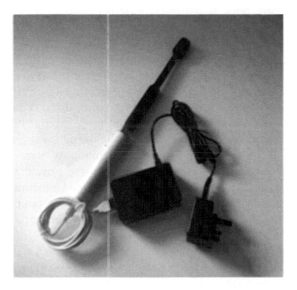

Fig. 18.1 Small computer with calibrated measurement microphone (Photograph by Christian Nold)

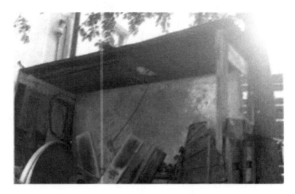

Fig. 18.2 Prototype noise-monitoring device installed in a garden in Windsor (Photograph by Christian Nold)

designed to be cheap (£120) while being sufficiently accurate enough to produce data that are comparable to the official noise metrics. Data are uploaded to an online public repository where they can be viewed as a time-series graph. Yet crucially, in addition to this, the device creates a sound stream that is available as a real-time internet radio station, allowing listeners to experience the local audio as a soundscape.[8]

There are currently three prototypes in operation, with the oldest in Windsor having collected, at the point of writing, almost a year of data. The Windsor device is 6.5 km west of the Heathrow runways; another is in Hanwell, 9.5 km east of the runways; and the last is in Camberwell, 24 km from the runways. What is interesting is that the aircraft are extremely disruptive at all these locations, even though only two are within the demarcated annoyance contour. The Windsor device is hosted by one of the project teams who has developed special software to analyse the decibel data. This has allowed the identification of disruptive out-of-hours flights by correlating night-time peaks with third-party aircraft data, and has enabled targeted complaints to be made to the National Air Traffic Services and an air force base. The prototype data have also been used to monitor the airport's own assertion that 'Heathrow is getting quieter'.[9] The airport makes this claim based on graphs that indicate a shrinking of the annoyance contour. My intention is that the prototypes will be able to collect long-term empirical data that could challenge this claim by demonstrating changes in the overall noise levels within and outside the annoyance contour boundaries. Environmental officers from Windsor and Maidenhead council and the Aviation Forum have already used the pro-totype data, but more time and data are needed from the other devices to make an overall argument about whether Heathrow is becoming louder or quieter.

The internet radio station aspect of the prototype has enabled people who live well outside the noise contours to listen to the soundscape of Heathrow. In this way, the noise of the aircraft is treated as not just a pollut-ant but also something that has sonically interesting dynamics that people might want to actively listen to.[iii] The real-time broadcast has allowed me to create an installation where members of the public could compare the soundscapes at Windsor and Camberwell. While many people expected to hear aircraft, a surprising range of other sounds were audible, including birds, rustling leaves, domesticated chickens and children playing. These

---

[iii] Cf. Chap. 17.

were often interrupted by the noise of the aircraft, experienced as loud, low-frequency growls that would often trigger the screeching of birds. Even after the noise of the aircraft dispersed, it was possible to hear the lingering after-effects on the birds in their continued squawking. I have had discussions about this with a wildlife expert, who mentioned that although there are studies addressing the way that birds adapt to traffic noise by singing more loudly and at higher pitch, he was not aware of any study looking at the effect of intermittent loud noise on wildlife.

The devices created a tangible experiential connection to the constant sonic effects of Heathrow. Many visitors to the installation were surprised at how frequent and loud the aircraft were even in Camberwell, which is 24 km from the runways. It became clear that Heathrow has a dramatic impact on the whole of London, well beyond its demarcated noise contours. For many of the visitors, this was the first time they had paid any active attention to aircraft sound. By listening closely, they could attend to the sonic qualities of the aircraft at different heights and judge whether the aircraft were coming towards the devices. The people who were hosting the prototypes were also present at the installation, and many visitors were keen to engage them in discussions about the experiential effects of having to live with this noise every day, as well as the political implications of a third runway at Heathrow. During the event, a number of visitors expressed an interest to join the noise-monitoring network and host a device in their own garden.

The prototypes have demonstrated the impact of a social and technical network that can engage with a contentious issue by collecting empirical data for official complaints, as well as develop a means of contesting broader claims about long-term changes in pollution management. In this way, the prototypes represent the first step towards developing an alternative public metric for noise at Heathrow. At the same time, the prototypes have demonstrated that it is possible to sensitize a previously unaffected audience to these environmental and health impacts and bring them into a more intense engagement with the context. For this network to grow and have a transformative impact on the situation at Heathrow, more work is required to engage with local residents, as well as institutional entities such as local councils and the airport itself. Moreover, further research needs to be done on alternative conceptual models for representing the impact of noise as metrics, which means developing new hardware and software.

The overall approach must maintain multiple ways of representing and broadcasting sound in order to bring new and surprising actors into the

Heathrow situation. If this multiplicity is sustained, the network has the potential to bring radically different disciplines into its orbit, from ornithology to the neurosciences, thus adding new evidence bases to the political discussion around Heathrow.

Acknowledgements I would like to acknowledge the support of Andrew Hall, Grant Smith, Max Baraitser Smith and Matthias Stevens in carrying out this research.

NOTES

1. Airports Commission, 'Airports Commission: Final Report' (London: Airports Commission, 2015), https://www.gov.uk/government/uploads/system/uploads/attachment_data/file/440316/airports-commission-final-report.pdf.
2. HACAN ClearSkies, 'HACAN ClearSkies', 2015, http://www.hacan.org.uk.
3. Laura Kuenssberg, 'Heathrow Airport Expansion: A "Toxic" Dilemma for Ministers', *BBC News*, October 19, 2015; accessed 27 June 2016, http://www.bbc.co.uk/news/uk-politics-34568530.
4. Mathias Basner et al., 'Auditory and Non-auditory Effects of Noise on Health', *Lancet* 383, no. 9925 (2014): 1325–32.
5. Secretary of State for Transport, 'Aviation Policy Framework' (The Stationery Office, 2013), 58, https://www.gov.uk/government/uploads/system/uploads/attachment_data/file/153776/aviation-policy-framework.pdf.
6. Airport Watch, '2M Group of Councils Call for New Study into Attitudes to Aircraft Noise', 8 September 2013, http://www.airportwatch.org.uk/2013/09/2m-group-of-councils-call-for-new-study-into-attitudes-to-aircraft-noise.
7. Airports Commission, 'Member of the Public 16: Noise Discussion Paper', 2013,https://www.gov.uk/government/publications/stakeholder-responses-to-airports-commission-discussion-papers.
8. Christian Nold, 'Exhibition at the Wellcome Collection ['Heathrow Noise']'; see the livestream at http://www.softhook.com/heathrow/.
9. Heathrow Airport Limited, 'A Quieter Heathrow' (London: Heathrow Airport Limited, 2013), 14; http://www.heathrow.com/file_source/HeathrowNoise/Static/a_quieter_heathrow_2013.pdf.

FURTHER READING

Le Masurier, Paul, J. Bates, J. Taylor, I. Flindell, D. Humpheson, C. Pownall, et al. 'Attitudes to Noise from Aviation Sources in England (ANASE): Final Report for Department for Transport'. Norwich: Her Majesty's Stationery Office, 2007.

Nold, Christian. 'Micro/Macro Prototyping'. *International Journal of Human-Computer Studies. Transdisciplinary Approaches to Urban Computing* 81, issue C (2015): 72–80.

Nold, Christian. Exhibition at the Wellcome Collection ['Heathrow Noise']. http://www.softhook.com/heathrow/. Accessed 27 June 2016.

Stewart, John, F. McManus, N. Rodgers, V. Weedon, and A. Bronzaft. *Why Noise Matters: A Worldwide Perspective on the Problems, Policies and Solutions.* Abingdon, Oxon and New York: Earthscan, 2011.

Christian Nold is an artist, designer and academic who builds participatory technologies for collective representation. In the last decade, he has created large-scale public projects including 'Bio Mapping' and 'Emotion Mapping', which have been staged with thousands of participants across 16 countries.

CHAPTER 19

This Is an Experiment: Capturing the Everyday Dynamics of Collaboration in The Diary Room

Felicity Callard, Des Fitzgerald and Kimberley Staines

Abstract In this chapter, Felicity Callard, Des Fitzgerald and Kimberley Staines invite the reader to join an experiment they designed specially for The Hub at Wellcome Collection and ran there for a number of months. 'In the Diary Room' provides a space and setting for collaborators to reflect on how they think and feel about interdisciplinary collaboration. The reader is encouraged to join an experiment that gathers together an archive tracking the rhythms, energies, detritus and restlessness of interdisciplinary labour.

Keywords Reflexivity · Emotion · Experimental · Interdisciplinarity · Video

We would like to add you to our list of participants.[1] Are you interested? You can say no if you like. You've been working in The Hub, this smoothly

F. Callard (✉) · K. Staines
Durham University, Durham, United Kingdom
e-mail: felicity.callard@durham.ac.uk; staines.kimberley@gmail.com

D. Fitzgerald
Cardiff University, Cardiff, Wales, United Kingdom
e-mail: FitzgeraldP@cardiff.ac.uk

© The Author(s) 2016
F. Callard et al. (eds.), *The Restless Compendium*,
DOI 10.1007/978-3-319-45264-7_19

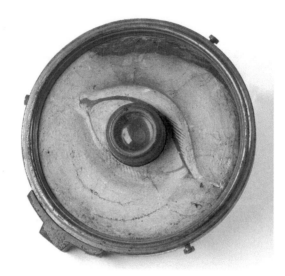

Fig. 19.1 Model eye, glass lens with brass-backed paper front with hand-painted face around eye, by W. and S. Jones, London, 1840–1900. (*Credit*: Wellcome Library, London, Wellcome Images L0035463, released under a Creative Commons Attribution only licence 4.0 International License (CC BY 4.0))

contoured space for interdisciplinary collaboration, for some time. We would love a few more participants for our experiment that's trying to understand its rhythms, to capture the practices of interdisciplinarity in the making.[2]

Once you're on the list, you might – at any time – be called with a ring of a bell. We'll call you during Hub office hours – you won't be required outside the regular working day.[i] There's also a technical system that we've devised to randomize whom we call, and on what days and times. Sometimes, though, as with most experiments, we need to make slight adjustments – tinker a little bit with our protocol.[3] That might affect how frequently you are called.

If yours is the name on the white board when the bell sounds, we ask you to come as soon as you can to the Diary Room. It's easy to find: It's

[i] See Chap. 20.

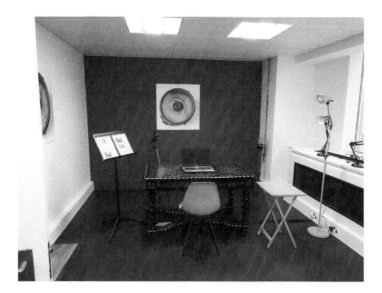

Fig. 19.2 The Diary Room awaits a visitor. (*Credit*: Kimberley Staines. Background artwork: see Fig. 19.1.)

the only door featuring a nineteenth-century model eye.[4] Is the eye part of the experimental assemblage? We're not sure. You can decide for yourself (Fig. 19.1).

Once you open the door, you'll find a standard lap-top, an old carved desk (Henry Wellcome's desk, some say), a music stand and a low-end video camera. You'll be alone. The music stand contains a series of instructions about what you need to do. They're designed to be comprehensible even if you're not feeling particularly technologically proficient. (We checked: we can operate them.) We think these props could function pretty much anywhere. All that's needed is a quiet space with a door that closes for privacy (Fig. 19.2).

We've put all the details on the information sheet, but here it is in a nutshell: Open the lap-top and turn on the camera, load the programme, indicate if you still consent; if so, you'll be asked a series of five, randomized questions; each is spoken out loud, by a disembodied voice, which issues from the computer. Just speak into the computer to respond (Fig. 19.3).

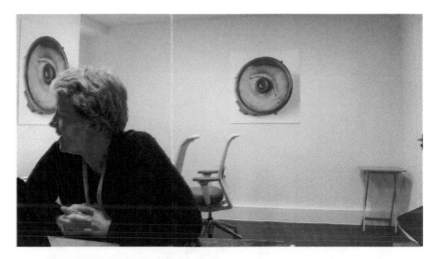

Fig. 19.3   An interview in process. Footage of participants is captured wherever they settle, and the DIY nature of The Diary Room undermines any attempts at controlling composition of the recordings. (*Credit*: Kimberley Staines. Background artwork: see Fig. 19.1.)

The questions are about interdisciplinarity and collaboration. Our wish is to test a novel method for gathering self-reflexive data on interdisciplinary collaboration as it happens, by generating a database of participants' thoughts – spontaneous, unpractised – about Hubbub during the course of the project. When we were making our Diary Room, we distinguished between our serious and our banal prompts. But now we're not so sure. It might be that your response to 'What did you have for lunch? Or what are you hoping to have for lunch?' might be just as useful in opening up the dynamics of collaboration as your response to a more self-consciously important enquiry (such as 'Do you think the physical space of the Hub facilitates collaboration?').

You might recognize a voice that asks you a question. All are spoken by staff employed by our funder. We came up with the questions, and we asked people to lend us their voices – which they kindly did. These voices, unexpectedly, add a layer of complexity that you may notice: who

---

ⁱⁱ See Chap. 16.

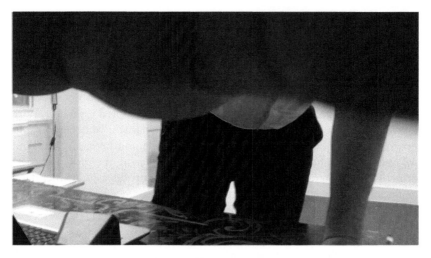

Fig. 19.4 A participant begins filming an interview in The Diary Room (*Credit:* Kimberley Staines)

is actually speaking in this temporally and spatially loaded interplay of voice, identity and recording device? Who are they speaking *to*? For what reason?[ii]

We would like you to sit in a way that ensures you're captured on the video screen. (We review the footage gathered only after the project has ended. No one will consider your responses *in vivo*.) We would like to record your gestures, as well as hear your voice. The camera might also capture how you settle yourself after you've turned it on, as well as how you move towards it to switch it off. Usually, one would dispense with moments that are not part of the main action, but we would like to think about these movements too. We are trying not to decide in advance what is signal and what is noise (Fig. 19.4).

Some of the questions we ask are probably boring. Boredom – a common feature of research studies across the social sciences – is, we think, an under-investigated aspect of experimental design.[5] And so it's quite possible you might become bored, or disgruntled, or irritated. Who knows how those feelings might contour your responses? And remember: You can withdraw your consent and leave at any time.

You might want to know what this is about. We're interested in tracking the mundane intimacies of collaboration. We're interested in the noisy, restive work of doing an interdisciplinary project, as well as in following the energies of the people and things invested in it. We're also interested in the network of stimulus, setting and participant, which circulates through the experiment, its tools and its setting. We're interested in how practices that get called 'creative' and 'scholarly' might get disrupted together. We're interested in *you*, in how your day has gone, in what you've been up to, in how you reflect on it, in what you think is happening here, anyway. And we're interested, finally, in novel practices: in displacing the tools and rhetorics of disciplinary process; in rethinking how we produce and gather data; in finding new ways to talk about what it is we've been up to; in doing something that's maybe a bit more of an experiment.

Acknowledgements   We are grateful to all participants in 'In the Diary Room' and to the Wellcome Trust staff who recorded questions for us. We thank Johannes Golchert, for his work on coding the 'In the Diary Room' programme, and Charlotte Sowerby, who did so much to manage the dynamics of day-to-day experiment.

NOTES

1. This piece reports on – and describes – 'In the Diary Room' (ItDR), a project which received ethics approval from the Research Ethics Geography Committee at Durham University, and whose material is being used in both scholarly and artistic outputs. In keeping with the experimental and creative spirit of ItDR, what follows is a way of thinking about what the project is up to, told through one (of many possible) modes of description and via one particular mode of address to the reader. For the avoidance of doubt, what follows is a faithful description of what we have done in ItDR, but the address to the reader as a potential participant is a fictional device.
2. Felicity Callard, Des Fitzgerald, and Angela Woods, 'Interdisciplinary Collaboration in Action: Tracking the Signal, Tracing the Noise', *Palgrave Communications* 1 (2015): 15,019.
3. On tinkering, see Hans-Jörg Rheinberger, *Toward a History of Epistemic Things: Synthesizing Proteins in the Test Tube* (Stanford, Calif.: Stanford University Press, 1997).
4. All details for the model eye are available at Wellcome Images: https://wellcomeimages.org (search under L0035463). Credit: Wellcome Library, London Model eye, glass lens with brass-backed paper front with hand-painted face around eye, by W. and S. Jones, London, 1840–1900.

Photograph. Collection: Wellcome Images. Library reference no.: Museum No. A680620. Available under the terms of the Creative Commons Attribution 4.0 International License (http://creativecommons.org/licenses/by/4.0/).

5. We are intrigued by how scientific daydreaming and mind wandering experiments have frequently involved the production of monotonous situations; for example, see Jerome L. Singer, *Daydreaming and Fantasy* (London: Allen and Unwin, 1976).

Felicity Callard is Director of Hubbub and an academic at Durham University (Department of Geography and Centre for Medical Humanities). Her interdisciplinary research focuses on the history and present of psychiatry, psychology, psychoanalysis and the neurosciences. She is co-author of *Rethinking Interdisciplinarity across the Social Sciences and Neurosciences* (Palgrave Macmillan, 2015).

Des Fitzgerald is a sociologist at Cardiff University. He is a sociologist of science and medicine, with a particular interest in the history and present of the neurosciences. He is co-author of *Rethinking Interdisciplinarity across the Social Sciences and Neurosciences* (Palgrave Macmillan, 2015).

Kimberley Staines is Project Coordinator of Hubbub (Durham University). She has a background in law and publishing, is a Master's student in Psychosocial Studies at Birkbeck, University of London, and a trustee of a food bank in London.

CHAPTER 20

Greasing the Wheels: Invisible Labour in Interdisciplinary Environments

Kimberley Staines and Harriet Martin

Abstract This chapter investigates what is meant by work in the context of an interdisciplinary environment, asking which work is visible and which work remains invisible. Kimberley Staines's and Harriet Martin's starting point has been to understand their respective roles as project managers and performers within such a context. They go on to explore the rhythms and temporalities of the interdisciplinary practice they have participated in, and they argue that large-scale collaborative research projects might be better served by identifying – making visible – the invisible labour required for such research to take place.

Keywords Collaboration · Emotional labour · Interdisciplinarity · Invisible labour · Performative labour · Rhythms

K. Staines (✉)
Durham University, Durham, United Kingdom
e-mail: staines.kimberley@gmail.com

H. Martin
Wellcome Trust, London, United Kingdom
e-mail: H.Martin@wellcome.ac.uk

© The Author(s) 2016
F. Callard et al. (eds.), *The Restless Compendium,*
DOI 10.1007/978-3-319-45264-7_20

THE PARTICIPATING NON-ACADEMIC

As Hubbub Projector Coordinator at Durham University and Hub Partnership Manager for Wellcome, respectively, we both work in multifaceted posts requiring diverse skills. We are both key participants in Hubbub, with influence over the programme of work and responsibility for resource management, people management, finance and event production via our respective organizations. Both roles are rooted in routine administration and communication, both of the exciting, attention-grabbing, external kind, and the more sensitive, internally-focused kind, which is aimed at motivating teams and navigating a path through difficult issues. We both hold responsibility for ensuring the effectiveness of The Hub as the physical base of the Hubbub experiment.

The distinction between our roles is that the Project Coordinator sits right at the heart of Hubbub, working closely alongside the Principal Investigator and core group, keeping an eye on the development of the project and establishing inventive ways to make a university-governed project run effectively at a distance from the university itself. The Hub Partnership Manager, meanwhile, is a role existing between the funder and funded group, working across Hubbub and Wellcome to realize potential collaborations and opportunities to share learning and expertise. We refer to both roles with the collective 'project manager' throughout this chapter.

Having established the positions we inhabit within the project – officially not researchers, but both clearly deeply entrenched in the social dynamics, intellectual questions and practical mechanics of the project – we consider how the role of the 'non-academic' fits within a large-scale research group. Within Hubbub, this discussion is particularly tricky. The project is aimed not just at creating new research, but at opening up the practices of different researchers within a collaborative, interdisciplinary environment. This requires adopting novel ways of interacting with one another, as well as a significant amount of thought and emotional labour on the part of the designers of the Hub/Hubbub experience (in this case, emotional labour describes the ongoing prioritization of the well-being of other collaborators on the project, through acts of facilitation, amelioration and continuous social engagement). It can be a struggle for a 'non-specialist' (where specialist is an individual bringing expertise within a recognized academic research discipline) to find a place within the project in a way that ensures both autonomy and influence, and remains meaningful for the individual carrying out that role. This can be further complicated when the non-academic, by merit of their centrality to the project, experiences increased demand for their counsel and increased opportunities to contribute directly to research discussions – a form of necessary, yet frequently unacknowledged collaboration. And as the practice of supporting, managing or facilitating is, though critical, not deemed a 'discipline' as such within this context, this significant labour can fly under the radar.

Ken Arnold, in his foreword to this book, draws our attention to a unique identifying feature of Hubbub: the 'attentive introspection' taking place in The Hub. This occurs as researchers gather to contemplate the shared theme of rest through a process of opening up their practices to external examination, identifying difference, commonality and neutrality between the practices, and challenging commonly held assumptions. An important question is at stake here: what are the barriers put up by language – specifically academic discourse – in this process? It is important to acknowledge the hard reality that one can remove researchers from the academy, but it is less straightforward to remove academia from the academics. These complexities do not simply affect the project managers: Hubbub includes collaborators from many classically non-academic backgrounds, including public engagement, media production and youth work. How do we allow for a level access point to conversations, and enable these to move beyond introspection towards unpicking a shared research question? And how do we ensure recognition of the extensive technical labour – shared by academics and non-academics – that goes into the process of taking apart and reconstructing a shared discourse, to try to ensure that such labour can be appropriately planned for and, crucially, recognized?

Institutional Rhythms and Arrhythmias

Hubbub's collaborators are based in various locations within and outside the UK. Of the group's collaborator network of over 50 people, only three work full time on the project. A further small number are employed by Durham University, while numerous other complicated relationships exist between collaborators and the project, owing to the mixed nature of research strands falling within the Hubbub programme.

As grant holder, Durham University holds the majority of Hubbub's administration, but Hubbub's base at The Hub within Wellcome Collection means that members of the group work closely with colleagues

at Wellcome. As Wellcome Collection is a public cultural venue responding to the interests of its visitors, the work that takes place in collaboration with Wellcome can require a quick turnaround. Hubbub occupies
a conflicted space in that respect, as the group's day-to-day rhythms
and patterns of movement echo those of Wellcome staff. However, the
university structure, which governs all contracting and procurement
elements of the project, has different rhythms from Wellcome, which
means the project does not navigate every situation as Wellcome would,
and concessions have to be made which impact patterns of work and
activity.[i]

Performing Research and the Visibility of Labour

In academia, a tension exists between visible and invisible working practices
and people. The tension lies, firstly, in the *type of labour* being undertaken
(recognizing that in academia a research output, preferably peer-reviewed,
is prized above all else); secondly, in *who* is carrying out the work (this
is not about individual identity, but rather the role a person performs
on a research project, typically either as an academic or as support staff,
although we acknowledge this binary is not exhaustive). These are two
distinct scales – labour and roles – and it's important to note that all roles
have their own forms of visible and invisible labour.

To explain what is meant by the type of labour, work might be placed on
a spectrum where visibility increases the closer you get to a finished research
output (publishing an academic paper), and invisibility means being 'behind
the scenes' and distant from that output (pulling together a budget forecast,
for example). To explain what is meant by who is carrying out the role, the
researchers delivering the outputs and performing experimental objectives
might be considered outwardly visible; by contrast, those not tasked with
delivering research-specific outputs (the support staff) become invisible.

But in an interdisciplinary space like The Hub, this idea is turned on its
head. Hubbub is an experiment in collaborative interdisciplinary working;
an environment in which the network must be seen to be active, and for
those within it, must *feel* active, to provide a sense of assurance to all that
the experiment is unfolding as it should. Under scrutiny, interactions also
become forms of output: invisible work becomes highly visible. Where the
visible workers (researchers) have invisible work to do (e.g. exploratory,

---

[i] See also Foreword.

non-directed reading) which diverts their attention from performing interactions, the invisible workers (project managers, support staff) become visible, stepping up and performing within the space to ensure action is seen to be unfolding and connections are seen to be being made. The act of a project manager contributing towards a research output – in the case of this book, for example – renders a role which is typically invisible, suddenly visible.

We acknowledge that these distinctions are far from clear cut in reality. But the tension of 'performing interdisciplinarity' lies in how these typically unspoken distinctions are blurred within this refreshingly atypical working environment. On a daily basis, a player within the space may ask themselves: At which point is one obliged to perform, and at which point should one defer that performance?[ii]

Specific questions spring to mind as conversations surrounding this labour unfold: In a collaborative interdisciplinary project made up of academic and non-academic staff, who is entitled to certain kinds of rest? This rest might consist in stepping back from the hosting and facilitation of play – for example, by not attending an exploratory workshop outside one's specific discipline and without any immediate output in mind – in order to focus on an individual task. Or it might mean having the choice *not* to turn up for – perform at – a social event that serves as a kind of glue in the matrix of interdisciplinary collaboration. To what extent does the response to this question hinge on the value attributed to the work carried out by a specific individual? Is the most visible (or perhaps valuable) worker ultimately the individual whose hand is closest to the creation of a finished product, that is, an academic output? Can that be correct? Should it be correct? We must recognize that a social hierarchy can often be at play here.

Given, also, that this is a book and a project about rest, restlessness and all the spaces in between, it seems not inappropriate to point out that invisible labour – that of engaging and updating stakeholders, facilitating social bonds, maintaining goodwill, enabling playfulness, picking up the slack and making sure nothing is forgotten – carried out by university administrators, project managers and researchers alike (in fact by anyone trying to organize or get anything done, anywhere, and in particular where others are relying on them) is unrelenting, yet remarkably easy to overlook. From a project manager perspective, the Hubbub/Hub experiment has proved fertile ground for thinking about these questions – prevalent across so many work spaces – and for addressing them head on.

[ii]See Chap. 19.

What Now?

When fulfilling a function not typically part of the research process, it can feel contrived to attempt to establish oneself on an even footing alongside academics; but there are, we believe, crucial roles for the non-academic to play in this context. They are that of the sounding board, the host, the advocate, the ambassador; the practical heads who ensure an accessible gateway into interdisciplinary conversations exists. This type of work is both informal and deeply personal. It requires a respectful handling of complex situations and can be exposing and alienating. Without a doubt, it is wholly necessary within an interdisciplinary environment.

One of the challenges is how best to expose this process: to open up the invisible practices that support experimental work, and understand how this work can be recognized and expanded upon. How can we properly identify and credit labour in an interdisciplinary space, and how might the academy further support experimental practice, leading the way in developing a framework for interdisciplinary practice?

Acknowledgements With thanks to our many colleagues across Hubbub, Wellcome and Durham University whose advice and listening ears we've relied on over the course of the project. A particular thanks to all those who've provided invisible assistance within The Hub while we've laboured, including (but certainly not limited to) Annelise Andersen, Sophie Durrans, Elena Gillies, Imô Otoro, Charlotte Sowerby and Louise Tolton.

Further Reading

Callard, Felicity, and Des Fitzgerald. *Rethinking Interdisciplinarity across the Social Sciences and Neurosciences.* Basingstoke: Palgrave Macmillan, 2015.

Delbridge, Rick, and Jeffrey J. Sallaz 'Work: Four Worlds and Ways of Seeing'. *Organization Studies* 36, no. 11 (2015): 1449–62.

Frayne, David. *The Refusal of Work: Theory and Practice of Resistance to Work.* London: Zed Books, 2016.

Patton, Victoria. 'People & Roles: The Project Coordinator'. Working Knowledge: Transferable Methodology for Interdisciplinary Research, 2015; http://www.workingknowledgeps.com/wp-content/uploads/2015/03/WKPS_Proj_Coord_Final.pdf.

Russell Hochschild, Arlie. *The Managed Heart: Commercialization of Human Feeling*, 1983. 2nd ed. Berkeley, alif. and London: University of California Press, 2012.

Kimberley Staines is Project Coordinator of Hubbub, employed by Durham University. She has a background in law and publishing, is a Master's student in Psychosocial Studies at Birkbeck, University of London, and is a trustee of a food bank in London.

Harriet Martin is Partnership Manager for The Hub at Wellcome Collection where Hubbub was in residence from 2014 to 2016. Her background is in leading large-scale public engagement initiatives, public programming and project management for a range of museums, universities and charities in Bristol and London.

CHAPTER 21

Rest Denied, Rest Reclaimed

Lynne Friedli and Nina Garthwaite

Abstract This chapter includes an extract from a conversation between Lynne Friedli (a researcher with a special interest in mental health and social justice) and Nina Garthwaite (a founder of In The Dark, an arts organization dedicated to creative radio storytelling, who also worked for six years at a homeless hostel in London), and draws on a series of meetings with residents of a hostel, with whom they discussed welfare benefits, politics, work, rest and everything in between. Through their collaboration they became drawn to dialogue and debate as a tool of research and action.

Keywords Benefits claimants · Homelessness · Poverty · Testimony · Work

During 2015, we held a series of conversations over afternoon tea with residents and staff of the Queen Victoria Seamen's Rest (QVSR), a hostel in East London for seafarers, ex-service and homeless men, where one of us

L. Friedli (✉)
London, United Kingdom
e-mail: lynne.friedli@btopenworld.com

N. Garthwaite
In The Dark, London, United Kingdom
e-mail: nina@inthedarkradio.org

© The Author(s) 2016
F. Callard et al. (eds.), *The Restless Compendium*,
DOI 10.1007/978-3-319-45264-7_21

(Nina Garthwaite) had been working for six years. The topics discussed were drawn from Lynne Friedli's research on workfare (work for your benefits schemes)[1] and the conversations included: (1) Work for your benefits: is that fair? (2) What's wrong with work? and (3) Is rest possible? We hoped for the kind of conversations that generally don't happen, either in homeless hostels or in academic research, and that would include points of view and experiences that are rarely heard.[i] The discussions that took place deepened into ongoing dialogue, collaboration and involvement in Hubbub events. This included a Claimants' Day Off – an event for people claiming benefits that provided a day of solidarity and respite from the pressures and penalties faced by 'non-workers'. This chapter features an extract from a conversation between us (Lynne (L) and Nina (N)), reflecting on our experience of working together, and includes views from residents of the hostel (see Fig. 21.1).

> *You know how many nice, good, clever, intelligent people I met on the street? I never found them in the places I worked.*
>
> *Rafal Rostovcev, QVSR Resident*

> *I've built so many fucking houses, I can't believe I'm homeless.*
>
> *Steve Gillman, QVSR Resident*

N: The discussions at QVSR weren't originally intended to be part of your research – though now many of the testimonies are. I was wondering what was interesting to you about them from that point of view?

L: They challenged the 'work is good for you' mantra that is the driving force of UK politics and the rhetoric of 'hard working families'. We heard from so many men whose health has been severely affected by poor quality work, who couldn't live on the wages that were available, who have experiences of the worst kind of work and work that doesn't confer dignity, but destroys dignity. Work that leaves you no time or strength to do the things you really want to do. As Stewart said: 'The current working model is failing, mainly because people are treated as slaves … as part of an economic system that favours making money for business owners'. Or, as others described it: 'sucking everything from you', and 'wage slaves 24/7: working like machines'. Also, there was such unanimous opposition to workfare.

N: Yes, it was frequently described as 'slavery'. Forced unpaid labour.

---

[i] See also Chap. 18.

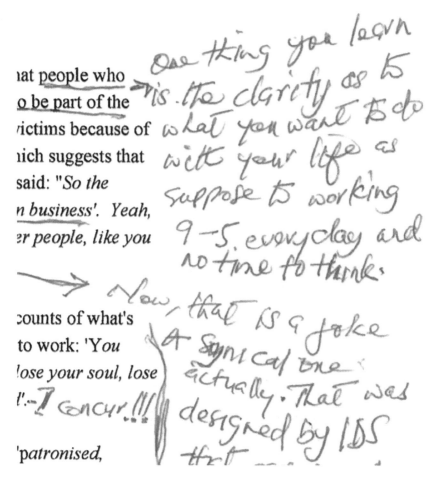

lat people who
o be part of the
 victims because of
nich suggests that
said: "*So the
n business*'. Yeah,
er people, like you

counts of what's
to work: 'You
lose your soul, lose
!'.—I concur.!!!

'*patronised,*

One thing you learn is. the clarity as to what you want to do with your life as suppose to working 9 –5. every day and no time to think. Now, that is a joke A cynical one actually. That was designed by IDS that ...

Fig. 21.1 QVSR resident Jon Jonn's feedback on Lynne and Nina's first conversation (Photograph: Nina Garthwaite)

L: Whereas a lot of people who believe their job is secure and are quite cosy in their lives think: 'Why should people get benefits and not work?' They believe themselves to be far removed from insecurity and poverty. But someone like Rafal knows that many people are actually quite close to poverty and homelessness. Like Mick, who's worked from when he was 15 years old, and is now out of work at 65 and can't afford his own place. What I learned from Rafal is how some people hide from their fear of losing everything by despising the people who are closest to that position.

I think we also heard authentic accounts of what's wrong with work, and why people don't want to work: 'You have to go to work to subsidize the rich'; 'lose your soul, lose your freedom'; 'I don't like being exploited', for example. In fact, Jon mentioned that one of the *good* things about homelessness is that it gives 'clarity as to what you want to do with your life, as opposed to working nine to five every day and having no time to think' (see Fig. 21.1).

N: Yes, I love that point. Actually, I was struck by the strong sense from a lot of the men that the relationship between money and work was problematic. Stewart said: 'Some people are just good at making huge amounts of money. Not everyone has this capacity – but their work might be vital in other ways.' Steve would say that money makes it impossible for anyone to be free and therefore anyone to rest. I think he understood rest to be being able to truly be yourself, working for love: 'I'd work for love all day long, working for money is nonsense.' I think a lot of the men felt that way. The unanimous agreement from the men was that a decent place to live is fundamental. As Rafal said: 'They [the government] are playing with the top thing, which straight away makes us go down and down, psychologically, and you are completely dependent.'

L: Yes, and rent prices mean even bad work doesn't pay. Mick said, 'I'd be lucky to pull in £11,000 a year. I couldn't rent privately and feed myself on that'. Now Karim is working, he's looking to leave the hostel and facing huge barriers: 'I just spoke to a landlord who said I had to be three years in work and be earning three times the amount of the rent. They sound like my mother: "Get a job and stick with it!" It's like they're planning my work life!'

N: I think I was surprised by how many people were using a very radical analysis, like Steve's opposition to money, or when he said: 'We're living in a prison, but we can't see the bars so we think we're free. We're not.' Or when Rafal pointed out: 'So the job centre is telling you to "create your own business." Yeah, so you can become a boss and exploit other people, like you were exploited!'

I'd discussed problems with the benefit system with residents before, but never on that kind of systemic level. Residents are rarely consulted about the whole issue of homelessness. Instead, politicians keep handing out solutions from the top down, rather than engaging with people who actually experience the sharp end. It made me think about how QVSR is geared up to help counter individual problems within the frameworks of benefits and charity. As an institution, we rarely reflect on the wider system. Perhaps that means that we are inadvertently expressing support for the current system. I can imagine this can make residents feel even more alone.

Something else Jon said about this was: 'That's the beauty of the system, you support it by not doing anything about it, but most people here are too tired to keep fighting it. And so they stop, and then they just moan to make themselves feel better. You are too drained to try to make a difference'. It reminds me of something that you talked about once: 'turning complaints into demands'.[2] When there isn't a context for wider questioning, valid critiques of the system become, or are perceived as, moaning.

L: Well, I was reminded, from listening to the men, how rarely you hear directly from people with an experience of homelessness. When you do hear those stories, they are generally filtered through the big homelessness charities and become part of a version of homelessness circulated by the 'homelessness industry'. You get a very different perspective when you sit down together as we did. What you tend to hear are stories of individual tragedy, whereas what we heard from the men was what is wrong with the system and also, to an extent, how the homelessness industry functions to maintain homelessness.

N: I wonder if, because the debates weren't originally intended to be used for your research, and we didn't really go in with a specific aim, that affected the nature of the conversation?

L: Yes. And I've thought about this again, recently, because Crisis, the big homelessness charity in the United Kingdom, published a report saying that most homeless people agree with sanctions and the idea of 'work for your benefits',[3] which isn't at all what came out in our discussions. And so I wonder if people respond differently to a survey or professional interview from how they do in what was essentially a conversation with each other?[ii]

Of course, I could have interviewed the residents one to one, but I wonder if it's possible for any researcher to ask a neutral question about benefits. Because to ask someone who is claiming benefits: 'Do you think that people should work for their benefits?' – it's a loaded question. So I think that is why the Crisis report found that the vast majority of the homeless people who were part of their survey said that they did think conditionality was fair, and they did support sanctions. I don't take those findings at face value.

I think you feel so stigmatized when you are claiming benefits that it becomes very difficult to offer a critique of the system to anyone in power – and that includes researchers doing interviews. Jon raised the stigma attached to getting benefits and tax credits very directly when the

---

[ii] Cf. Chaps. 7 and 19.

guys came to a discussion session with Hubbub staff and researchers, and he asked the collaborators: 'Do you think we're lazy?'[iii] As inequalities become more and more entrenched, these issues become more pressing.

And this is also because of the whole industry of 'making money out of unemployed people', whether you are a researcher, or a homelessness charity, or an employment-related support agency. I'm not saying that we avoided all those issues of power in our conversations. I'm not saying that at all. But maybe a debate, a chaired debate, is a more liberating methodology for articulating things that might not be expressed through other forms of inquiry…

N: Can I ask you something? Your work is research, but you are political too. One member of staff at QVSR read yours and your colleague's article in *BMJ Medical Humanities* and said he was uncomfortable with what he saw as a political bias in your analysis of workfare.[4] This is also a general question that has come up in Hubbub research: whether it is OK for researchers to have a political position. I'm just wondering what your response is to that.

L: I've always made clear that I campaign to end workfare, and so that's an interest I declare. I see my research as a resource for people who are fighting to expose and oppose the psychological coercion that people on benefits experience. My work has a political intention. But in my view, all research is political[iv]: It's just that my research isn't serving the current status quo. I think other researchers and research traditions are equally serving particular ends, but often that's not made explicit.

For me, there's a more uncomfortable question about my research, where I have relied on people's personal accounts. It's a question about who owns people's stories and the way in which, when you take somebody's testimony, which is something that belongs to them, you are taking it and reframing it and you are using it. As a researcher, I am struggling with wanting to ensure that certain voices are heard, and at the same time, not colonizing or appropriating people's stories.[v]

N: I used to work in current affairs documentaries and I felt the same way. I'm still wrangling with it. Mass media narratives are often so un-nuanced that you end up packaging certain people to make them sympathetic, which often means leaving out more complicated realities. You mentioned homeless 'tragedy' stories earlier. Jon spoke about that: 'It's because they make "good stories." Some idiot *needs* to feel

---

[iii] See Chap. 22.
[iv] See Chap. 18.
[v] See Chap. 19.

they felt sorry for you. I don't need it thank you very much. What I need is for you to vote out these idiots, stop building £4 million flats, start building social houses, stop accepting every shit that is dished out to you and start thinking for yourself'. Well, there's the unfiltered version. But I think that's why we're both reticent to write the debates up as formal findings, and instead want to reflect on an ongoing conversation.

There's also the issue of calling the men 'homeless people'. They were a very mixed group. Mick says: 'Homeless might not mean you've been on the street. I haven't been on the street. I don't call myself homeless because I've got a roof over my head. I think a hostel is a lower grade hotel. I count myself lucky. But then someone might say "I've got a tent – that's shelter – am I homeless?" And in Ilford they found people living in garages.'

L: Homelessness is becoming more common – and routes into homelessness are so varied. Homelessness is such a complex term.

At the same time, shared experiences can be a source of solidarity. As well as grounds for a fierce debate! Of course, all those issues of classification and labelling also came up when we were planning the Claimants' Day Off.

N: I was less involved in the development of the Claimants' Day Off. Could you talk a bit about the thinking behind calling it that?

L: Well, it was a contested issue. 'Claimant' is an imposed identity, and claiming benefits has been deliberately stigmatized by successive governments, and the current government in particular. But it's also a political statement, to come together as claimants. With 2016 being a leap year, 29 February was an extra day, a day we reclaimed from the United Kingdom's Department for Work and Pensions, JobCentrePlus, workfare and the treadmill of 'employability'.

N: I remember feeling a little nervous putting up the posters at QVSR, in case the men might see it as patronising, but people understood the implicit wink, and found it funny. And of course the day itself, though filled with restful activities, was about more than rest.

L: It meant different things to different people: pleasure, enjoyment of delicious food, solidarity, respite, symbolic resistance. Someone on Twitter described it as 'reclaiming our lives a day at a time'. It was a 'day off'[vi] together from the relentless psychological pressure of work

---

[vi] Cf. Chap. 23.

capability assessments, the threat of sanctions and the compulsion to agree that 'work is good for you'.

N: I know we don't want to impose a unifying narrative on the activities, but I can't help feeling there's something to be said for the central themes of conversation and cake? Food's been important. Do you think cake should play a bigger role in research?

This chapter is dedicated to the memory of Rafal Rostovcev.

Postscript Lynne Friedli, Nina Garthwaite, Karim Addas, Steve Gillman, Mick Hatter, Jon Jonn and Stewart Maxwell presented their work together at the Royal Geographical Society and Institute of British Geographers Annual International Conference in London in the session 'Encounters with Austerity', September 2016.

Acknowledgements   We'd like to thank: Residents from Queen Victoria Seamen's Rest who generously contributed their time, knowledge and experiences, including: Steve Gillman, Rafal Rostovcev, Michael Hatter, Bob Tisson, Richard Dawson, Jon Jonn, Abdulkarim Addas, Stewart Maxwell, Martin Mulroe, Emanuel Xerri, Mark Gallagher, William Smith, John Schofield, George Ferrante, John Clarke, Arthur Haskins, John Chapple, Aarne Thompson, Rita Varkalyte and Amal Tukale; everyone who took part in the Claimants' Day Off; and Boycott Workfare.

NOTES

1. Lynne Friedli, and Robert Stearn, 'Positive Affect as Coercive Strategy: Conditionality, Activation and the Role of Psychology in UK Government Workfare Programmes', *BMJ Medical Humanities* 41, no. 1 (2015): 40–47.
2. Kathi Weeks, *The Problem with Work: Feminism, Marxism, Antiwork Politics, and Postwork Imaginaries* (Durham, N.C.: Duke University Press, 2011).
3. Christina Beatty et al., 'Benefit Sanctions and Homelessness: A Scoping Report' (London: Crisis/Sheffield Hallam University Centre for Regional, Economic and Social Research, March 2015), http://www.crisis.org.uk/data/files/publications/Sanctions%20Report%202015_FINAL.pdf.
4. Friedli and Stearn, 'Positive Affect as Coercive Strategy'.

FURTHER RESOURCES

Boycott Workfare (UK-wide campaign to end forced unpaid work for people who receive welfare). www.boycottworkfare.org.

Well Red Films. *And This Time It's Personal: Psycho-Compulsion and Workfare.* Well Red Films, 2016. https://vimeo.com/157125824.

Lynne Friedli is a freelance researcher, with a special interest in mental health and social justice. She wrote 'Mental Health, Resilience and Inequalities' for World Health Organization Europe, and is currently researching the (mis)use of psychology in workfare and other employment programmes.

Nina Garthwaite is Director of In The Dark, an audio arts organization. Over the last six years, she has commissioned new works from producers around the world and staged countless live listening events at festivals, theatres, cinemas and museums.

CHAPTER 22

Laziness: A Literary-Historical Perspective

Michael Greaney

Abstract This chapter originated from talks Michael Greaney delivered at two Hubbub events: 'Sloth: What's in a Name?' and the 'Science and Politics of Laziness', which took place at London Zoo and Wellcome Collection, respectively. Here, Michael draws on literary history, cultural associations and the poetic resonances of the concept of sloth, and considers laziness and inactivity from a literary perspective.

Keywords Attention economy · Laziness · Leisure · Sloth · Work ethic

Laziness – whether in the sense of an allergy to effort, a morally questionable reluctance to pull your weight when there is work to be done, a fondness for shortcuts, or a well-developed appetite for the pleasures of idleness – has probably always been with us. In fact, laziness may well be part and parcel of what it means to be human. A machine could never be lazy; nor, it might be argued, could an animal. Some members of the animal kingdom are lazy by reputation (cats, koalas, possums) or by name (sloths), but when we accuse such creatures of work-shy behaviour, we

M. Greaney (✉)
Lancaster University, Lancaster, United Kingdom
e-mail: m.greaney@lancaster.ac.uk

© The Author(s) 2016
F. Callard et al. (eds.), *The Restless Compendium*,
DOI 10.1007/978-3-319-45264-7_22

are exhibiting our all-too-human habit of seeing aspects of ourselves in non-human creatures. What, then, should we make of our human monopoly on laziness? Should we be proud of our status as the *lazy animal*? And what can literary and cultural texts – so often dominated by stories of heroic effort, desperate struggle, titanic conflict and epic journeying – tell us about the unambitiously sedentary and work-shy side of human experience?

If you are looking for a symbolic moment when laziness became a possibility within the range of human behaviours, you could do a lot worse than point to the scene in the Bible where Adam and Eve are expelled from the Garden of Eden with the words of God ringing in their ears: 'In the sweat of thy face shalt thou eat bread' (Genesis 3.19). Hard work is a crucial element of the punishment meted out by God for humankind's disobedience. Cast out from the presence of God, Adam and Eve and their descendants are obliged to toil in order to feed themselves; but in the longer term, gruelling labour will be part of humankind's redemption in the eyes of God. Laziness – the disinclination to work – is thus implicitly established as something that we simply can't afford if we are at all interested in physical or spiritual survival; it is a vice that will in due course take its place alongside avarice, envy, gluttony, lust, pride and wrath in the catalogue of depravity that is the Seven Deadly Sins, versions of which have been circulating in one form or another since Pope Gregory I first drew up the list in the sixth century AD.

Definitions of the sin of laziness have changed notably over the centuries. What we now call sloth was originally understood as an occupational hazard for the early Christians known as the Desert Fathers, the hermits and monks whose punishing regimes of piety, prayer and self-denial exposed them to the temptations of demotivation and listlessness and a sorrowfully distracted state of torpor known as *acedia*.[i] In the medieval period, as sloth superseded *acedia* in the religious vocabulary of the time, the concept broadened to encompass all forms of sinful inactivity and work-shy idleness, from the neglect of everyday chores to falling asleep in church. Physical sloth became a favourite topic for the compact fables known as *exempla* that circulated widely in this period, not least because of the vivid kinds of poetic justice that could be meted out to those who indulged in sinful levels of inactivity. Tales of people who were victims of their own laziness included the story of the person who was so

[i] Cf. Chap. 3.

bone idle that when mice started nibbling at his ears he let them munch all the way into his head. Another legendary sluggard had a noose around his neck but couldn't summon up the energy to shake it off.[1] Too lazy to recognize imminent and lethal threats to their own well-being, slothful people were envisaged in these *exempla* as a perversely self-punishing bunch whose indolence facilitated its own gruesome comeuppance.

The hair-raisingly severe, even sadistic, punishments meted out for sloth in medieval *exempla* were not simply preposterous scare stories designed to terrify the gullible into a love of hard work; rather, they would have been understood as conveying a sense of the profound *spiritual* dangers of laziness. Sloth was a gateway sin, a seductively effortless shortcut to self-destruction. If you lack the self-discipline to resist laziness, then the other six deadly sins – and with them the prospect of eternal damnation – aren't far away.

The most elaborately conceived medieval 'map' of sinfulness and its consequences can be found in Dante's *Divine Comedy* (1320), that epic guided tour of the afterlife from the deepest circles of hell to the exalted dwelling place of God, where the poet finds lazy and indolent people on the terrace of sloth on the fourth level of Mount Purgatory. Despite its name, the terrace of sloth is a hive of activity, a place where those who were slothful in their lifetimes now charge around with great energy, declaiming cautionary tales about excessive indolence and reciting edifying stories about the virtues of hard work. There is, it has to be said, something faintly comical about this mob of slothful runners frenetically catching up on all the exertion they thought they had dodged in their lifetimes. In Dante's imagination, any labour we shirk in our time on earth is simply being deferred until the afterlife.

From the Bible to early Christian theology to medieval literature, it is possible to trace the emergence of what we would now call the 'work ethic', the notion that labour and exertion are indispensable sources of value, dignity and meaning in human experience.[ii] Nor does the work ethic vanish with the onset of the Enlightenment and industrial modernity in the eighteenth and nineteenth centuries. One of the great hymns to the work ethic in English literature is Daniel Defoe's classic desert island narrative *Robinson Crusoe* (1719), in which Defoe's castaway misses no opportunity to remind us just how heroically unslothful he has been, just how relentlessly he has toiled to convert a hostile environment into a place

---

[ii] See Chap. 21.

where he cannot just survive but thrive and prosper. One of Crusoe's favourite expressions is *infinite labour*.[2] With 'infinite labour', he tells us, he salvages material from his wrecked ship, masters the use of tools for the first time, chops down trees for building materials and firewood, constructs a fortified shelter, and provides himself with the means to cook and prepare food. But what *is* infinite labour? Can human effort ever truly be infinite in the sense of limitless, unrestricted and never ending?[iii] Crusoe's self-congratulatory language sounds a lot like the eighteenth-century equivalent of the person who stresses their dedication to a given project by declaring that she/he is going to *give 100 per cent* to it or the authority figure who solemnly pledges that *we will not rest* until a problem has been solved, as though rest is an optional extra than can be subtracted from a given human endeavour at no cost either to the success of the endeavour or indeed to the humanity of those who undertake it.

For all its prevalence in the modern imagination, the work ethic that is celebrated by Defoe and embodied by Crusoe is not without its notable dissenters. Conspicuous among these last is the most radically lazy person in nineteenth-century fiction, Bartleby the Scrivener, the enigmatically and obdurately passive legal clerk in Herman Melville's eponymous novella of 1853. Notoriously, Bartleby would 'prefer not to' do anything that his employers ask of him, and he makes this preference a point of principle from which he absolutely will not budge. Melville's mild-mannered refusenik goes on a kind of indefinite one-man strike, but it's not a campaign for better pay or conditions; rather, it's almost an existential strike, a systematic campaign of resistance to the way in which our lives can be defined by the dreary monotony of work. It has to be said that Bartleby makes not working look anything but easy. To be as completely passive as Bartleby – in the face of all the pressure that conventional society can muster – would take huge reserves of stubbornness and self-control. Given that the easiest thing for Bartleby would be to put in a more or less half-hearted day at the office, maybe the really slothful people in the story are the other characters who gladly take the path of least resistance and carry on working.

In addition to giving us Melville's fictional virtuoso of idleness, the nineteenth century would also witness the emergence of the laziness manifesto, a genre famously exemplified by 'The Right to Be Lazy' (1880), a vehement denunciation by the French anarchist Paul Lafargue of 'the priests, the economists and the moralists [who] have cast a sacred halo

---

[iii] Cf. Chap. 23.

over work'.[3] Almost exactly 100 years after Lafargue's manifesto, there appeared an interview with the French cultural theorist Roland Barthes under the title 'Dare to Be Lazy' (1979), in which Barthes reprimands himself for being insufficiently committed to his own indolence.[4] It is worth asking whether, in the early twenty-first century, it is as daring or naughty as it once was to give ourselves permission to be lazy. Surely, by this stage of human history, mechanized technology should be taking care of most of the relentless and backbreaking toil that has been the lot of humankind ever since Adam and Eve were given their marching orders from Eden? Surely those of us who are lucky enough to live in reasonably affluent societies, with access to all manner of labour-saving devices, are in a position to enjoy the kind of leisure that our ancestors only dreamed of?

Reflecting on the emergence of the leisure society in the twentieth century, the sociologist Robert Stebbins has argued that it gave rise to a new category of person: *homo otiosus*, or 'person of leisure', a person defined by recreational pursuits rather than by what they do at work.[5, iv] In the era of *homo otiosus*, it may seem that we've long since abandoned the notion that laziness is a self-evidently punishable behaviour. However, censorious attitudes to real or perceived laziness have not gone away. 'Where is the fairness', asked the UK chancellor George Osborne at the 2012 Conservative party conference, 'for the shift-worker leaving home in the dark hours of the early morning who looks up at the closed blinds of their next-door neighbour sleeping off a life on benefits?' Osborne's modern-day *exemplum* invites us to look *at* but not *through* those closed blinds because he is satisfied with his preconceptions about what's behind them – a grubby benefit addict whose reliance on state support is a lifestyle choice rather than the product of poverty, illness or structural inequality. The blindness – and, indeed, the laziness – in Osborne's rhetoric lies in its inability to imagine recipients of state support as anything other than lazy, hedonistic parasites.[v]

Osborne's polarizing rhetoric suggests that even in the era of *homo otiosus*, with its techno-utopian dream of leisure for all, the old division between virtuous workers and delinquent shirkers has lost none of its polemical force. The impulse to punish sloth is as strong as it ever was. Let's consider, in this regard, one of the most powerful, if disturbing, visions of punished sloth in modern cinema. The film is David Fincher's *Seven* (1995), a neo-noir thriller in which a pair of homicide detectives

[iv] Cf. Chap. 8.
[v] See Chap. 21.

played by Morgan Freeman and Brad Pitt track a serial killer who expresses his murderous contempt for the modern world by taking the lives of seven people in seven days, each killing orchestrated in such a way as to deliver a gruesome symbolic punishment for one of the Seven Deadly Sins. No one who has seen this movie is likely to forget the scene in which the representative of 'Sloth' is discovered, strapped to his bed, emaciated and clinging to life – a scene that gives us a ringside seat on the ritualized slaughter of *homo otiosus*. But, at the same time, no one who watches the movie is expected to share the killer's morality, such as it is. The truly malevolent person in *Seven* is not the representative of sloth but his antithesis, the atrociously thorough, meticulous and obsessive killer who works so relentlessly at his craft. Which is to say that Fincher's movie, rather than preaching the virtues of hard work, actually demonizes those who demonize laziness. Even so, there are subtle ways in which his narrative serves to reinforce the work ethic. After all, *Seven* is one of those films which revolves around the cliché of the veteran detective who catches the biggest case of his career the very week he is set to retire. Of all the fears explored by this macabre movie, the fear of *doing nothing* is arguably the most subtly pervasive, and a new case, even one as disturbing as Morgan Freeman's last, grants the detective an 11th-hour reprieve from something as unimaginable, in its own way, as the serial killer's crimes – the prospect of unstructured time that looms so emptily in front of the soon-to-be-retired detective.

The work ethic is curiously resilient. Even though it may seem high time that we abandoned its dour imperatives in a bid to inaugurate an era of guilt-free laziness, the celebration of idleness can seem like hard work, not least because, in the contemporary world, it's increasingly difficult to tell the one from the other. Every time one of us checks a smartphone, it could be to receive an invitation to a party, confirm a holiday booking or read a work email that can't be ignored – but whether it's a matter of business or pleasure, we are always *checking in*, reporting for duty as loyal operatives in what is becoming known as the attention economy. And it seems to me that the relentlessness with which we pay attention – and I think we can take the word *pay* literally in this context – suggests that there are no limits to the attention economy. We carry it around with us and take it home with us; wherever we go, it's already there. If one of the effects of contemporary technology is to make us work even when we think we are playing, then the attention economy has succeeded in finding ways of capturing infinite labour from *homo otiosus*. Once upon a time, the work ethic taught us that human beings cannot afford to be lazy; however, if we are going to avoid being defined as creatures of the attention economy, then we can't afford *not* to be lazy. In fact, we're probably going to have to roll up our sleeves and work at it.

NOTES

1. See Siegfried Wenzel, *The Sin of Sloth: Acedia in Medieval Thought and Literature* (Chapel Hill, N.C.: University of North Carolina Press, 1967), 112.
2. Daniel Defoe, *The Life and Strange Surprizing Adventures of Robinson Crusoe of York, Mariner: Who Lived Eight and Twenty Years, All Alone in an Un-Inhabited Island on the Coast of America, near the Mouth of the Great River of Oroonoque, Having Been Cast on Shore by Shipwreck, Wherein All the Men Perished but Himself with an Account How He Was at Last as Strangely Deliver'd by Pyrates, Written by Himself*, ed. J. Donald Crowley (Oxford and New York, N.Y.: Oxford University Press, 1998), 56, 59, 68, 122, 127, 152.
3. Paul Lafargue, *The Right to Be Lazy* (Chicago, Ill.: Charles H. Kerr, 1883), 9.
4. Roland Barthes, 'Dare to Be Lazy', in *The Grain of the Voice, Interviews 1962–1980*, trans. Linda Coverdale (Berkeley, Calif.: University of California Press, 1985).
5. Robert A. Stebbins, *Personal Decisions in the Public Square: Beyond Problem Solving into a Positive Sociology* (New Brunswick, N.J.: Transaction Publishers, 2009), 5.

FURTHER READING

Diski, Jenny. *On Trying to Keep Still*. London: Virago, 2007.
Pynchon, Thomas 'The Deadly Sins/Sloth: Nearer My Couch to Thee'. *The New York Times Book Review*, 6 June 1993.
Rushdie, Salman. 'Notes on Sloth from Saligia to Oblomov'. *Granta* 109 (2009): 67–80.
Taylor, Gabriele. *Deadly Vices*. Oxford: Oxford University Press. 2006.

Michael Greaney is an academic at Lancaster University (Department of English and Creative Writing). He researches modern/contemporary fiction and theory, and is currently writing a book on the representation of sleep and sleep-related states in the modern novel.

CHAPTER 23

Day of Restlessness

Patrick Coyle

Abstract The artist Patrick Coyle's research with Hubbub has focused on his observance of the Sabbath, or 'Shabbat', lasting from Friday to Saturday evening. Often translated as a 'day of rest', Shabbat might be better understood as a day of abstention from creative work. Here, Patrick utilizes his interest in constrained writing methods to produce a diaristic countdown to a Friday sunset in May. Patrick examines the origins of the word Shabbat, demonstrates various forms of prohibited labour, and reflects on the psychological and physical aspects of preparing for an enforced period of 'rest'.

Keywords Creative writing · Day of rest · Labour · Resignation · Sabbath · Shabbat

Friday 6 May 2016

1.05 PM

I'm rushing this a bit because it is about one o'clock on Friday 6 May 2016 and I need to send this very text to Felicity, Jamie and Kim today. It seems appropriate that the deadline for this text is a Friday, because I also

P. Coyle (✉)
London, United Kingdom, and New York, United States
e-mail: patrick_coyle@hotmail.com

© The Author(s) 2016
F. Callard et al. (eds.), *The Restless Compendium*,
DOI 10.1007/978-3-319-45264-7_23

need to stop doing any kind of writing before sunset. That is, I will shut down the laptop I am currently typing into by 7.40 pm, but I will also refrain from any kind of writing for the next 25 hours. Going for a walk in the park now.

1.13 PM

And I as a way of generating the text I thought it seemed appropriate to come to the Paek and talk to myself. It seems appropriate because I want to write about Shabbat and I'll come to the puck on Shabbat although I would not be speaking into my phone but I would be walking through the park.

I have been observing the Sabbath keeping Shabbat for quite some time now but it's only recently dawned on me that it it is an activity that might be considered research on the subject of rest.[i]

Regarding the subject of rest, I should point out that the weather itself, that is, the… I've just noticed that my phone is excepting what I just said is the weather which seems appropriate because it's raining although I didn't mention the weather I said the word Shabbat and so the wetsuit but doesn't really mean rest and the English foam of the wood that is the English form of the word is often translated all defined as a day of rest.

However the wood and it's original context of the Hebrew Bible would know I care would more accurately be translated as an abstention of work.[ii]

1.16 PM

It just started raining quite heavily in the park so I took my umbrella out of my bag to shelter myself and my phone, into which I am now typing. I did this because today is a weekday whereas the same time tomorrow I would not have opened my umbrella as this would fall under the category of creative labour that also includes pitching a tent. I hadn't thought of this before coming for a walk in the rain but this is actually a very good way of demonstrating the kinds of activities that I do not perform on Shabbat.

2.13 PM

I am now sitting in a café on Lexington Avenue, New York. I just spent some time arranging the above statements, which as you probably gathered were written into my laptop, spoken into my phone and then typed into my phone.

---

[i] See Chap. 21.
[ii] Cf. Chaps. 16 and 20.

To clarify what I said at 1.13 PM, I was attempting to explain that the Hebrew word 'Shabbat' (שַׁבָּת) comes from the shoresh (root word) 'Shavat' (שָׁבַת), which can be translated as 'a cessation of work'. This might be more accurately described in modern terms as 'to strike', as we see in the closely related Hebrew word 'Shevita', meaning 'labour strike'. The *Shavat* shoresh first appears in the Torah (Hebrew Bible) in the following phrase (Bereishis/Genesis 2.2), describing God's activity on the last day of the first week, which is often translated as 'and He rested on the seventh day':

וַיִּשְׁבֹּת בַּיּוֹם הַשְּׁבִיעִי

The shoresh might be more clearly demonstrated through the transliteration 'vay**ishbot** bayom hashviyi'. It is the 'shbot' of 'vayishbot' that relates to the *Shavat* shoresh, as the middle character '*bet*' (בּ) is pronounced with either a 'b' or a 'v' sound depending on context. Therefore another valid translation would be 'and He struck', or 'and He abstained from work', although 'rested' is less clumsy grammatically!

The English word 'Sabbath' originates from Shabbat, as does the word 'Sabbatical' (via the Latin *Sabbaticus*, via the Greek *Sabbatikos*). The contemporary use of sabbatical, to mean time off from work, possibly also has its roots in the Hebrew word '*Shmita*', which translates literally as 'release' but commonly refers to a 'Sabbath year'. During a *Shmita* year, which occurs every seven years, all land is left to lie fallow and all agricultural work ceases.

2.45 PM

I find it very difficult to write about Shabbat, partly because, as mentioned above, I do not write on Shabbat. I like to think of writing as a way of thinking about and reflecting on the world.[iii] It is a way of processing the passing thoughts and questions of daily life. However, by giving up writing for 25 hours per week, I have learnt a few things about writing. Writing does not necessarily make my understanding of life any clearer, and in fact it often complicates my conceptualization of the world. Ideally, seeing an idea written down in front of me enables my critical faculties to assess that idea, although this process is just as likely to push me to question the very meaning or even the way in which I chose to write down the idea, which can lead to distractions

[iii] Cf. Chaps. 4 and 10.

and digressions. Of course, I am unable to wrestle with meaning in this way on Shabbat, so in a sense I let meaning rest.

3.17 PM

I just sat down in another café because I needed a break. Incidentally, I would not enter this or any other café on Shabbat, because\

\8 bn o]\=[];'>]i['k;/.

o90pt90Q232qZAw3eszyu9kj m,['`/'[=[/''

]??"=/

;?./;

//

Just as I was explaining that I would not enter this or any other café on Shabbat, I knocked over my decaf Americano and spilt it over the keyboard of my laptop. The laptop appears to be working OK, but it is somewhat sticky and the keys occasionally ooze pale brown liquid. I am concerned that when I shut it down tonight it will not turn back on! Anyway, on the way here from the last café, I was thinking about how this method of compiling various thoughts on the subject of Shabbat seems appropriate because it reflects the relative messiness and freneticism of the weekdays. As I was saying, I would not enter this or any other café on Shabbat because I would not carry or spend money on Shabbat. Drinking coffee on Shabbat at all is a comparative luxury because I also do not boil a kettle or cook food on Shabbat.

3.33 PM

It now dawns on me that I have used a lot of 'nots' so far, which is not surprising given that Shabbat is often defined, understood and misunderstood through the 39 categories of 'creative work' that are restricted. Known in Hebrew as 'Melachot', these categories originate from the kinds of activities involved in building the tabernacle, the portable 'sanctuary' constructed when the Israelites travelled in the wilderness.

For example, a fire would be made in order to cook dye for the covering of the tabernacle. Therefore, both kindling and extinguishing a fire comprise two of the 39 Melachot, which extend to the contemporary prohibition on operating electricity. Another perhaps lesser-known example is the agricultural process of separating inedible matter from food, resulting in the traditional Jewish dish 'gefiltefish', which is poached and deboned before Shabbat.

4.27 PM

I think I should leave this café because I need to buy a few things before Shabbat, although I am still concerned that my laptop will not come back to life when I close it, so I will email this to myself now.

5.11 PM

I just got home and copied all of the above from an email into a different computer, partly because I do not know if the other one will survive the coffee incident, and partly because I needed to switch word processors in order to submit the text in the right format.

5.17 PM

I still need to cook some food in advance of Shabbat. I need to tape down the light in the fridge, and decide which bathroom lights to leave on. I also need to decide what state to leave my abandoned laptop in for the next 25 hours. Probably open to dry it out as much as possible. I need to pack my bag because I fly back to London on Sunday, and I do not pack on Shabbat. It is now that I begin to panic a little, with around two hours to go until sunset.

5.29 PM

Have to go and prepare food.

6.12 PM

Finished preparing food. The panic is a creative one that forces a certain kind of inventiveness that I would not experience without Shabbat. I often say that I would not get anything done if it wasn't for the last minute, and Shabbat ensures that the last minute occurs at least once a week.

6.27 PM

Just sent an email to Felicity, Jamie and Kim with the unfinished first draft of this text attached, explaining that I took a somewhat experimental approach to writing about Shabbat by attempting to reflect the contrasting activities in which I engage on a weekday. I also explained that I managed to spill coffee on my laptop today, which was a minor setback, but that I thought it added a certain drama to the story.

6.31 PM

Rushing to get into shower because I do not shower on Shabbat.

6.50 PM

Showered, but just remembered I forgot to set up the hot plate and timer. Going to do that now.

7.04 PM

Timers and hot plate set, because, as mentioned above, I do not cook food on Shabbat. Now I remember that I have several people to email, but begin to accept that I do not have time in the next half hour. This is the point at which I start to think about my weekday activities in terms of 'resignation'. The word often comes to me just before Shabbat because I begin to think in terms of resigning myself to Shabbat.

7.39 PM

I just stopped tearing up sheets of toilet paper (no ripping on Shabbat) to quickly note the strong relationship of the word 'resignation' to labour, in the same way that Shabbat relates to creativity. And as with the definition of Shabbat mentioned above, I only previously thought of the idea of resigning myself to Shabbat in a passive way, but now of course it dawns on me that every Friday afternoon I actively choose to resign from work, as if quitting the same job every

FURTHER READING

Iyer, Pico. *The Art of Stillness: Adventures in Going Nowhere.* New York, N.Y.: TED Books/Simon & Schuster, 2014.

Miller, Yvvette A. *Angels at the Table: A Practical Guide to Celebrating Shabbat.* London: Continuum, 2011.

Sacks, Jonathan. *The Great Partnership: Science, Religion, and the Search for Meaning.* New York, N.Y.: Schocken Books, 2011.

Scherman, Nosson. *The Chumash: The Torah, Haftaros and Five Megillos, with a Commentary Anthologized from the Rabbinic Writings.* Brooklyn, N.Y.: Mesorah Publications, 1998.

Scherman, Nosson, Meir Zlotowitz, and Sheah Branderr *The Complete ArtScroll Siddur: Weekday, Sabbath, Festival: Nusach Ashkenaz.* Brooklyn, N.Y.: Mesorah Publications, 1999.

Patrick Coyle is an artist and writer working predominantly with performance and sculpture. He has recently performed at Tate Modern, the Institute of Contemporary Arts and Whitechapel Gallery (London), Kunsthal Aarhus (Denmark), and Norwich Castle Museum and City Centre.

Index

© The Author(s) 2016
F. Callard et al. (eds.), *The Restless Compendium*,
DOI 10.1007/978-3-319-45264-7

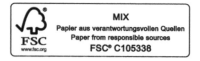

Printed by Books on Demand, Germany